Atopic Dermatitis - Essential Issues

Edited by Celso Pereira

Published in London, United Kingdom

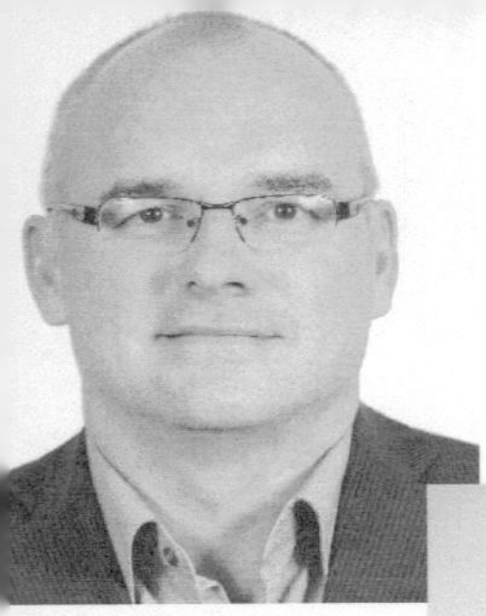
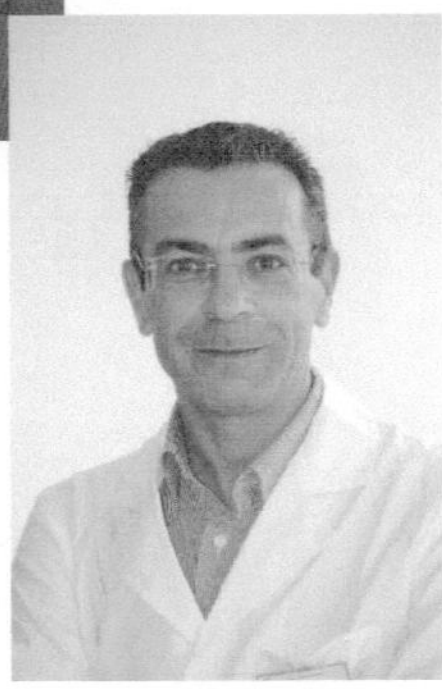
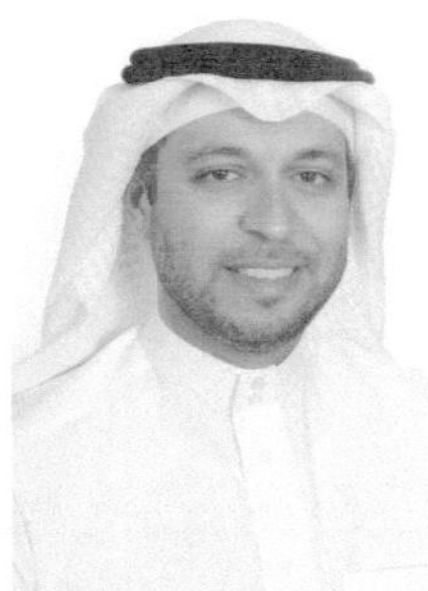
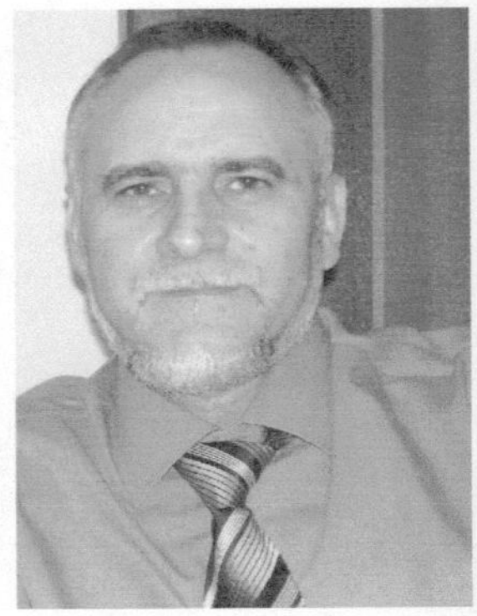
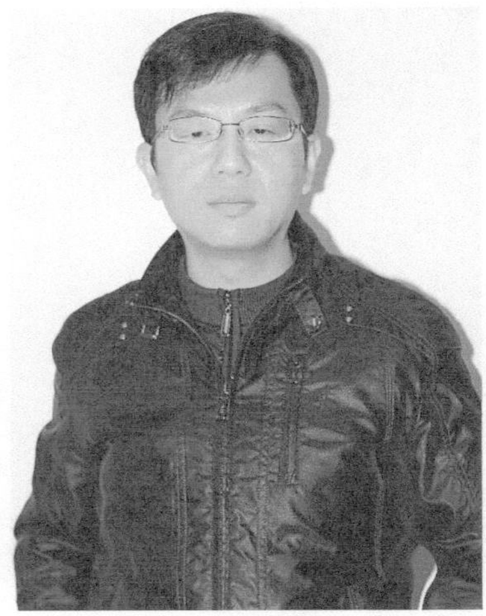
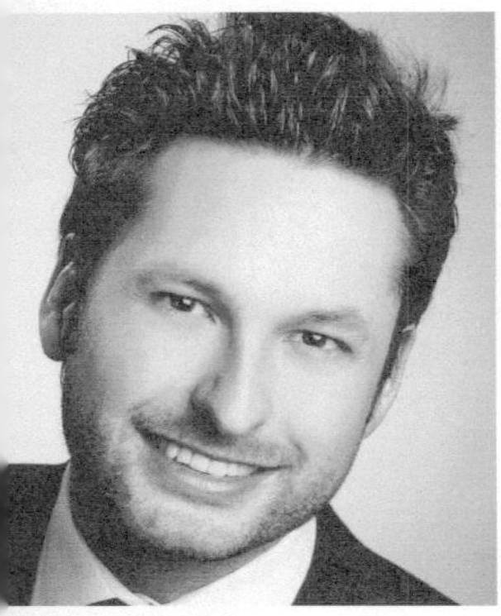
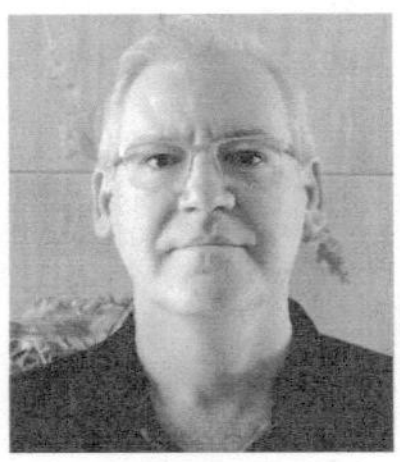

IntechOpen

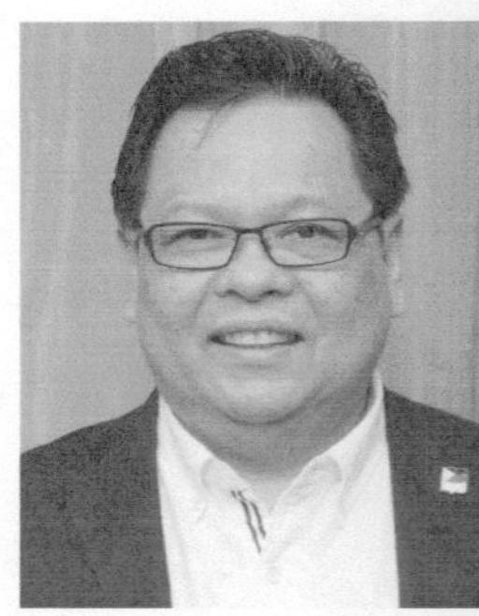
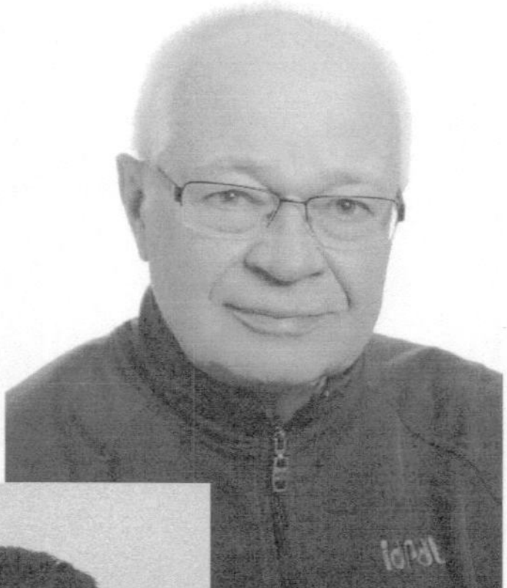
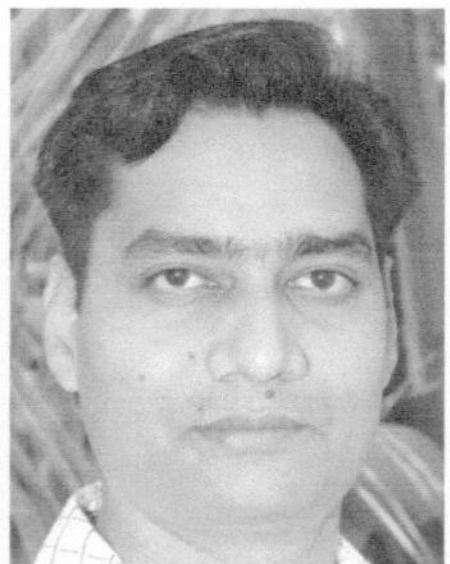
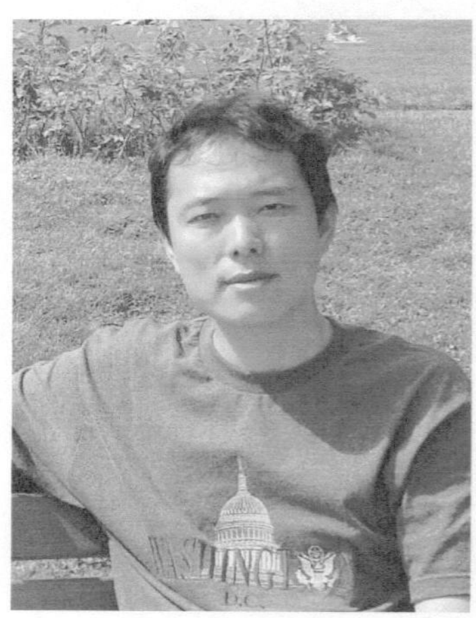
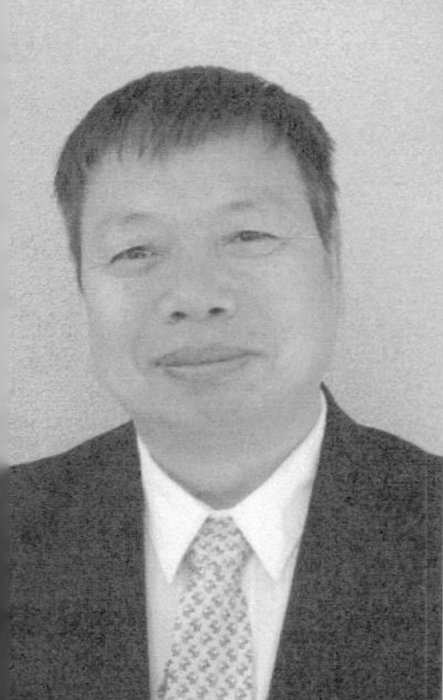
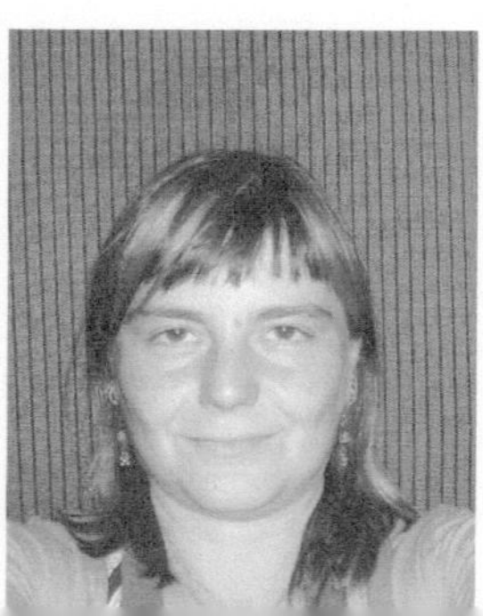

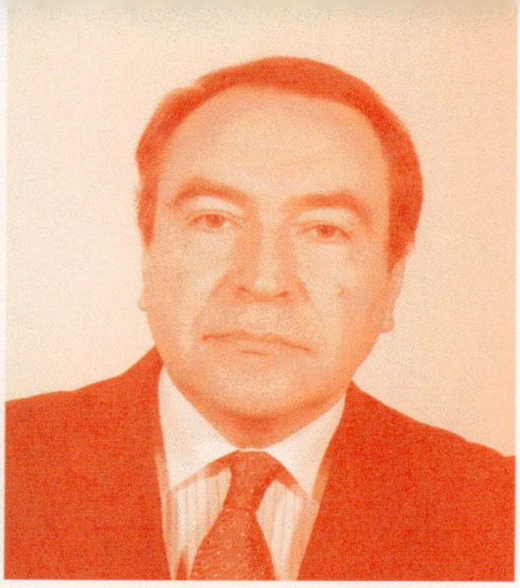
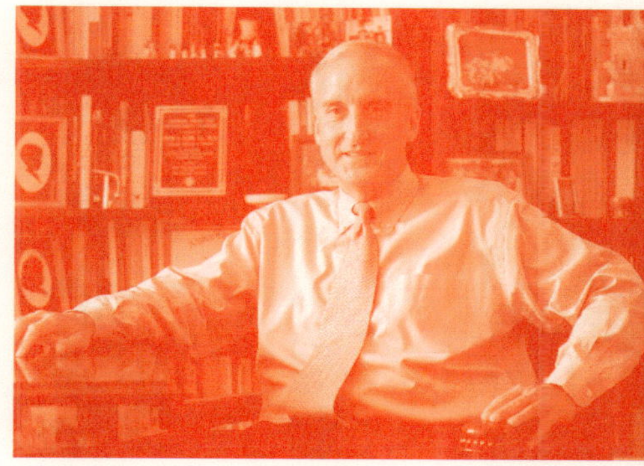
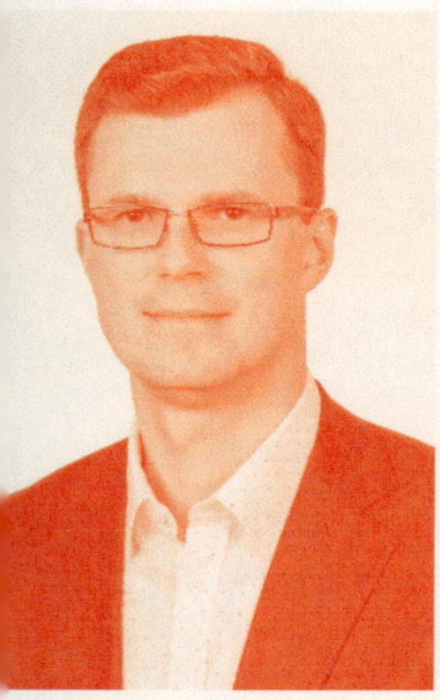
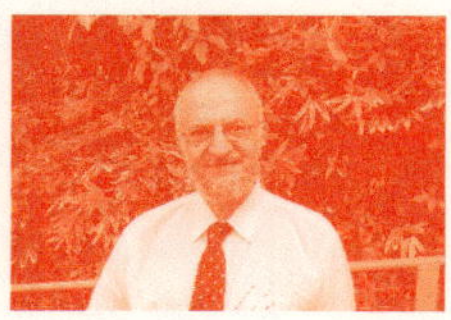
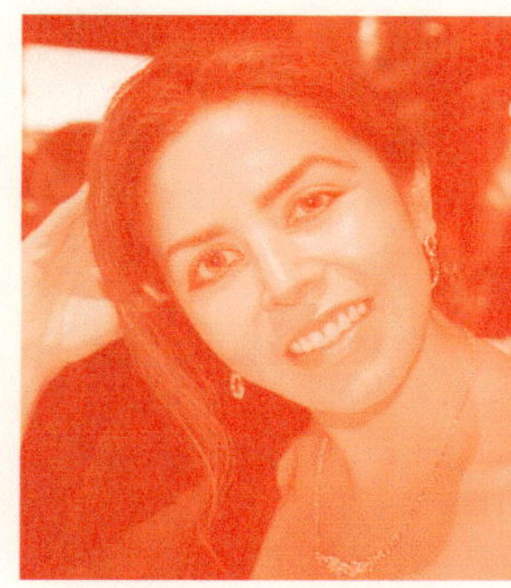

Supporting open minds since 2005

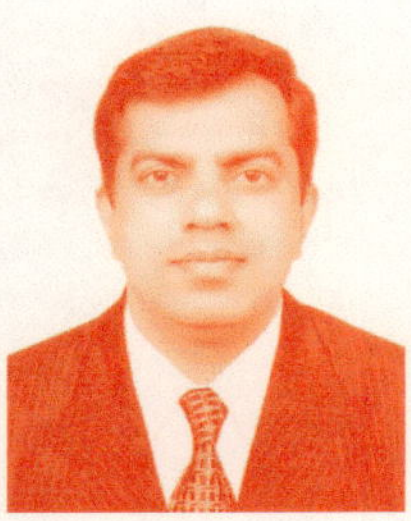
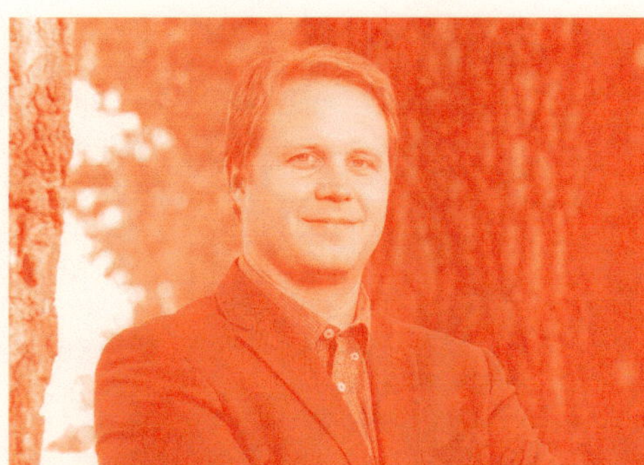
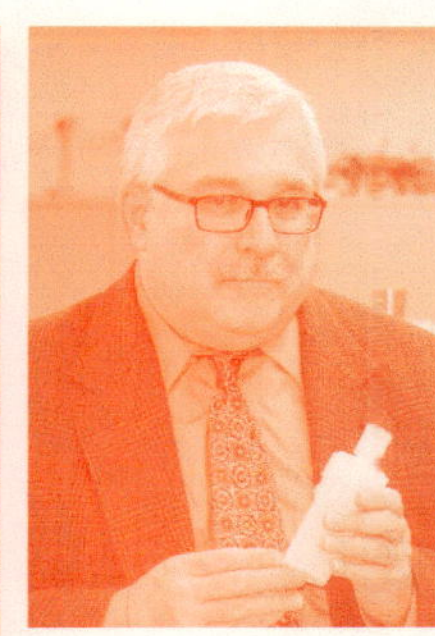
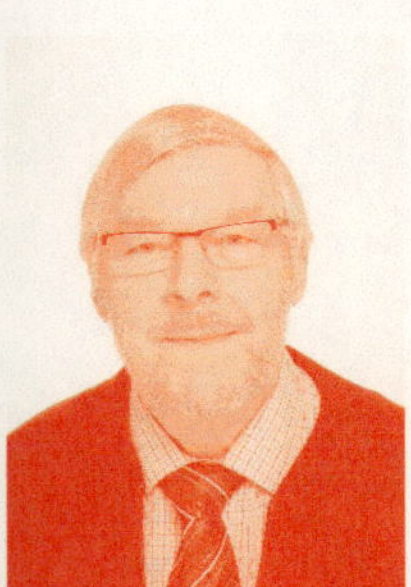
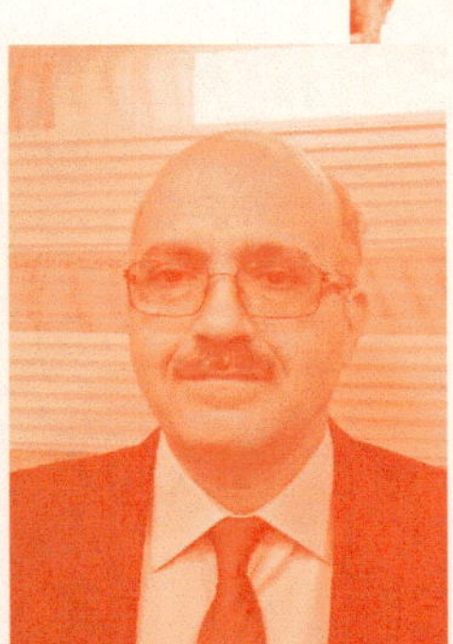
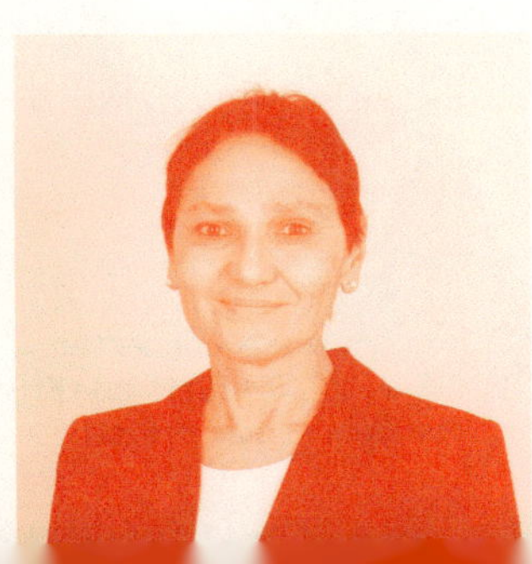
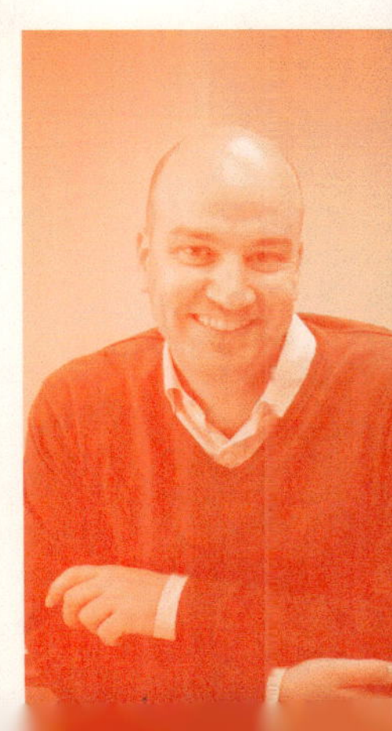

Atopic Dermatitis - Essential Issues
http://dx.doi.org/10.5772/intechopen.91492
Edited by Celso Pereira

Contributors
Ignasi Figueras-Nart, Oscar Palomares-Gracia, Ivana Filipovic, Milan Lackovic, Zorica Zivkovic, Slađana Mihajlovic, Tamara Bakic, Đorđe Filipović, Suvarna Samudrala, Aleksandra Lesiak, Joanna Narbutt, Magdalena Ciazynska, Joel Noutakdie Tochie, Mazou Ngou Temgoua, Gael Ananfack, Vladimir Sobolev, Elizaveta Bystritskaya, Oxana Svitich, Olumayowa Abimbola Oninla, Ayesha Omolara Akinkugbe, Mufutau Murphy Oripelaye, Fatai Olatunde Olanrewaju, Bolaji Otike-Odibi, Celso Pereira

First published in London, United Kingdom, 2021 by IntechOpen
IntechOpen is the global imprint of INTECHOPEN LIMITED, registered in England and Wales, registration number: 11086078, 5 Princes Gate Court, London, SW7 2QJ, United Kingdom
Printed in Croatia

British Library Cataloguing-in-Publication Data
A catalogue record for this book is available from the British Library

Additional hard and PDF copies can be obtained from orders@intechopen.com

Atopic Dermatitis - Essential Issues
Edited by Celso Pereira
p. cm.
Print ISBN 978-1-83962-723-1
Online ISBN 978-1-83962-724-8
eBook (PDF) ISBN 978-1-83962-735-4

For EU product safety concerns:
IN TECH d.o.o., Prolaz Marije Krucifikse Kozulić 3, 51000 Rijeka, Croatia, info@intechopen.com or visit our website at intechopen.com.

Meet the editor

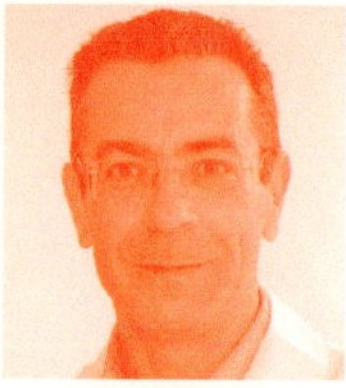

Prof. Celso Pereira, MD, Ph.D., is head-chief of the Clinical Immunology Unit and Clinical Herbal Medicine in Clinical Practice, Medicine Faculty, Coimbra University, Portugal. He is also a specialist in immuno-allergy at Coimbra's University Hospital Centre, Portugal. He was the past president of the Immuno-allergy Board of the Portuguese Medical Association. His main activities include clinical practice, education (pre and postgraduate) and clinical and laboratory research. He is a member of national committees on vaccination, diagnostic procedures in allergy and immunology, and monitoring hypersensitivity reactions to COVID vaccines. Dr. Pereira is also a coordinator of some clinical guidelines approved and under application by Portuguese health authorities. Nowadays his scientific interests include research in the mechanisms of respiratory allergy, specific immunotherapy, and applications of medicinal plants.

Contents

Preface

Atopic dermatitis is one of the most common skin disorders, particularly in children. The enormous heterogeneity of mechanisms, triggers, clinical severity patterns, and treatment strategies have contributed to a huge set of data that allows for more personalized management of this condition. In fact, research has identified several clinical phenotypes and precise pathogenic mechanisms.

In addition to the standard pharmacological, topical, and systemic treatments, new anti-inflammatory, immunomodulatory, and biological agents are currently undergoing clinical trials with very promising results, despite the lack of clinically robust biomarkers. This book presents the most current physiopathogenic evidence in atopic dermatitis and the scientific rationale of the currently available therapeutic arsenal as well as new options for treating severe forms of the disease. Written by experts in the field, chapters address some of the most current particularities in atopic dermatitis.

I am convinced that the information contained herein will allow for better management approaches to patients with this condition as well as instigate and appoint new lines of research. I would like to thank all the contributors and the staff at IntechOpen for making this project possible.

Celso Pereira
Clinical Immunology,
Medicine Faculty,
Coimbra University,
Portugal

Chapter 1

Introductory Chapter: The Multispectrum Faces of Atopic Dermatitis

Celso Pereira

1. Introduction

Atopic dermatitis is a chronic or recurrent inflammatory skin disease usually related to the atopic march and atopic morbidity. Although the onset of symptoms occurs predominantly at pediatric ages, the disease can start at any age and even the elderly.

A constellation of conditioning factors has been identified, most of them sustained by genetic and epigenetic aspects favoring a Th2 cell profile, intrinsically associated with many other factors of the skin itself, namely the localized immunoinflammatory responses, the skin barrier dysfunction, dysbiosis, neuroimmune dysregulation and obviously environmental determinants and many others conditions [1]. As a consequence, different phenotypes and endotypes result from multiple heterogeneous and complex pathogenic mechanisms that are clinically expressed with different levels of severity and in the specific location of the lesions [2].

At pediatric ages, the thickness of the skin is markedly reduced compared to adults, as well as the population and diversity of resident cells [3]. In case of skin inflammatory disease the homeostatic disruption on cells as well on the matrix structures determines intrinsic changes in the skin's adaptive immunity facilitating an inducible skin-associated lymphoid tissue (iSALT) with critical consequences [4].

The microbiome has a particular interest in all medical areas and aim of profuse scientific interest in the last decade. However, it was the results of the Sanford study that surprisingly came to prove the magnitude and diversity of cell-free DNA in our body [5]. In fact, the placental microbiome is decisive in the fetal period. So, gut and skin newborn microbial flora is markedly dependent on the maternal clinical condition and the type of delivery, eutocic or instrumented [6, 7]. However, the postnatal period, depending on intrinsic and exogenous factors, will allow the acquisition of new microorganisms. It therefore occurs a process of specialization in niches, and the subsequently interaction with the host comes to allow functional differentiations in this own flora having obvious consequences on mucosal structures [7].

The skin microbiota in the healthy individuals is highly variable between designated areas of moist, such as the surfaces of the antecubital and popliteal fossae, and areas of naturally drier skin or sebaceous skin areas, particularly regarding the proportions of the *Phyla Actinobacteria, Firmicutes, Proteocbacteria e Bacteriodetes* [8].

Dysbiosis in atopic dermatitis resulting from increased expression of *Staphylococcus genera*, particularly *S aureus* species, has been consensual for a

IntechOpen

long time and the acute outbreaks had been frequently described corroborate this increase with a parallel decreases in *Streptococcus* or *Propionibacterium* species [9]. The overexposure in the skin of *S aureus* and, less frequently to *Malassezia furfur*, results on environment specific conditions that favor a local immunoinflammatory hyperactivation in opposition to the protective effect of *Acinetobacter* species [10].

Atopic dermatitis also has an apparent correlation between the intestinal axis and the cutaneous mucosa, with over-expression of *Clostridium difficile* and *Faecalibacterium prausnitzii* species, reduction of short-chain fatty acids metabolites, which may enable future and potential extra-cutaneous therapeutic implications [2, 9, 11, 12].

This recent data amplify the complexity of the pathophysiology and immunological mechanisms in atopic dermatitis already accepted, namely: the skin barrier dysfunction, the type 2 inflammatory immune response and other important cell axes such as the dependents of cell ways Th22, Th1, Th17 or *JAK–STAT* signaling pathway [13].

The enormous complexity of pathways and mechanisms involved in atopic dermatitis is based on a huge heterogeneity of polygenic determinisms, so the genome-wide association studies (GWAS) only allow confirming the heritability identification in a very limited number of patients. The best documented gene mutation is related to filaggrin, but is only present in around 30% of the European population [14]. Concerning skin barrier dysfunction other genes has been also described (loricrin, keratin-16 periplakin e *SPINK5/LEKTI*), but it requires more research to assess the magnitude and prevalence in a large patients samples studies [2]. Likewise for a typical type T2 inflammation the dysfunctions of IL-4 and IL-13 *loci* are also far from being present in all patients [2].

Pruritus is one of the hallmarks of atopic dermatitis and can have a dramatic and severe impact on the quality of life of patients at all ages. From a clinical and pathophysiological point of view, the pruritus induced by histaminergic pathway is not a standard feature in opposition to other atopic diseases. In addition to the classic inflammatory type T2 cytokines (IL-4 and IL-13), the IL31 and, to a lesser extent, TSLP, are strictly related to pruritus signaling, particularly in severe forms. Despite the presence of IL-4Rα in afferent neural fibers, these neural structures also have IL-31Rα receptors, activated by the release of this cytokine by T2 cells, but also by mast cells, dendritic cells and activated keratinocytes [15].

Thus, pruritus is, rather than a clinical sign dependent on the inflammatory process, but itself an active intervening part on the pathogenic mechanism, allowing increased keratinocyte IL-31 release by damage and scratching, and also an increased activation of dermal dendritic cells via TSLP. Symptomatic control is, therefore, decisive, in terms of the immense discomfort experienced by the patient and also because allow a negative feedback to the underlying skin inflammation [13].

In the light of the above, inhibition of IL-4Rα receptors by dupilumab allows for a significant control of pruritus thresholds in a very expressive number of patients. However, in others, this control is not achieved. Trials with nemolizumab, an anti-IL-31Rα monoclonal, look like it is highly effective in controlling itching, but with significant clinically adverse effects [15].

In an interesting experimental model with human mast cell lines, an alcoholic extract of *Commiphora myrrha* reduced not only the release of histamine, but also the production and release of IL-31 by kinase suppressor regulated by an extracellular signal and activation of *NF κB* [16]. If these results are confirmed *in vivo*, this essential oil could have an enormous impact in the routine clinic associated with a reduced burden economic impact.

The treatments currently recommended by different guidelines and consensus from different international scientific societies are strictly guiding in pharmacological and non-pharmacological care plans, namely: general measures, hydration to minimize barrier defects, topical treatments, systemic anti-inflammatory drugs for specific conditions and biological treatment for severe forms. Naturally, many of the new therapies are very expensive, which limits their access to many patients around the world [2, 13, 17].

However, several articles have pointed out other strategies that appear to be promising and highly elective in atopic dermatitis.

Emollients are essential to care, and it has been suggested an additional inclusion of ceramides or plant extracts with anti-inflammatory activity, despite the need for robust evidence [18–20].

Regarding anti-inflammatory therapy, the different classes of corticosteroids, calcineurin inhibitors and an inhibitor of the intracellular enzyme phosphodiesterase 4 represent the drugs currently available for topical treatment. Inhibitors of the *JAK–STAT* and tyrosine kinase pathways are currently in clinical trials. Delgocitinib (a pan-*JAK* inhibitor) has recently been approved in Japan for the treatment of adults with atopic dermatitis [2, 21].

Regarding systemic therapy it is recommended to severe presentations of atopic dermatitis, and in recent years it has been seen a profusion of new approaches with new biological drugs, some of them already available and many others in clinical trials [22, 23]. This topic is developed in a specific chapter in this book.

The spectrum of action of these new drugs, targeting glycoproteins (IgE), cytokines, chemokines (or their receptors), cell signaling pathways and cell surface receptors, should be submitted to a extensive drug-safety monitoring and rigourous pharmacovigilance programs, because most of them are generally ubiquitous in multiple cells, tissues and organs and could have potential uncontrolled consequences, even in short-term treatments. In addition, this profusion of new drugs is not accompanied by biomarkers that allow a specific selection for different phenotypes and endotypes, in a pathology as heterogeneous as atopic dermatitis.

The new data that comes from the knowledge of dysbiosis in atopic dermatitis must be consistent with new research lines. These findings will allow new therapeutic approaches in earlier stages and more primary pathophysiological conditions that support the immune-inflammatory process and support the chronicity and clinical severity.

The presence of cutaneous biofilms in severe clinical forms and with skin recurrent infections and impetiginization has extremely relevance on the clinical point of view [24]. Current treatment strategies do not establish nor allow the elimination of these structures on the skin surface. However, a growing number of *in vivo* and *in vitro* investigations have demonstrated that topical extracts of some medicinal plants had the ability of biofilms dysruption from bacteria (*Staphilococcus spp* e *Streptococcus spp*) or fungi (*Malassesia furfur* and *Candida spp*) [24, 25].

Like many other chronic conditions in which dysbiosis is subject to extensive research, also in allergic diseases and atopic dermatitis in particular, several studies sustain that in the treatment plan new approaches will be necessary, some of which with very promising *in vitro* and *in vivo* results [26]. There are countless potential manipulation and modulation possibilities of dysbiosis, but additional studies are still necessary to prove the efficiency and safety criteria [27].

Topical application of bacterial lysates or bacteriophage-derived enzymes seems to be one of the most feasible strategies. This strategy tends to, selective, replace strains considered commensal identified on the skin of healthy individuals or others comproved strains with competing effect for *S aureus* [27]. Another researches address the topical application of non-replicating probiotics that may allow a negative modulation in the viability of dysbiotic bacterial flora [28].

Bacterial lysates administrated sublingually have been in clinical use since the 1970s, for the prevention of infectious risk in respiratory pathology. Resulting from lysis of heat-inactivated bacterial strains, the composition can be selected and adjusted to a very diverse number of strains [29]. Without an obvious reason, its use in the clinic was markedly decrease in the late 1990s, but it has recently been a subject of interest and rediscovery given the potential of the mechanisms of action. In this context, the designation of "trained immunity-based vaccines" has been proposed since these vaccines allow effects on both innate and adaptive immunity [30, 31]. Among the most relevant mechanisms are the antimicrobial cytokine response, overexpression of TLRs; production of specific IgG and induction of regulatory T responses and regulation of dendritic cells [31]. In patients with strongly impetiginized forms, there is the possibility of personalized prescription with one extract containing strains adjusted to dysbiosis. This formulation administred at sublingual region, adjacent to the MALT structure, is highly promising from an immune point of view, compared to the oral formulas, which is usually restricted to formulations and fixed compositions of lysates [32].

Other potential treatment strategies involve the autologous bacterial transplant, allogeneic bacterial transplant or even fecal microbial transplantation. On these grounds, further and roboust research is necessary [33–35].

Likewise, well-designed studies are needed to define the position and the role of probiotics, prebiotics or symbiotics in atopic dermatitis. This subject is developed in a chapter of this book, as well the specific criteria for phototherapy in select patients.

In view of the enormous clinical heterogeneity, of the physiopathological mechanisms, the treatment of atopic dermatitis is a real concern over the opportunities and therapeutic options already available and all other strategies under development and trials [2, 16–23, 36, 37].

So, nowadays the atopic dermatitis treatment is a real challenge in view of the enormous clinical heterogeneity, the physiopathological mechanisms, the immunogenic aspects and the tremendous variability regarding age, race and ethnicity [37].

In this context, the opportunities with the available therapeutics and all the other strategies under development will certainly allow us to increasingly personalize the management plan and in a future that is believed to be close the identification of robust biomarkers for phenotypes and endotyps, as also on monitoring approach.

The scientific review of some of these aspects in the chapters of this book will certainly be tools of great interest and importance in the knowledge of a pathology with colossal prevalence and a tremendous impact on the quality of life of these patients and their families.

Author details

Celso Pereira
Clinical Immunology, Unity; Herbal Medicine in Clinical Practice, Unity; Medicine Faculty, Coimbra University, Coimbra, Portugal

*Address all correspondence to: celsopereira.pt@gmail.com

References

[1] Paller AS, Spergel JM, Mina-Osorio P, Irvine AD. The atopic march and atopic multimorbidity: Many trajectories, many pathways. The Journal of Allergy and Clinical Immunology. 2019;**143**(1):46-55

[2] Langan SM, Irvine AD, Weidinger S. Atopic dermatitis. Lancet. 2020;**396**(10247):345-360

[3] Saitoh A. Aizawa Y2 Sato I, Hirano H, Sakai T, Mori M. skin thickness in young infants and adolescents: Applications for intradermal vaccination. Vaccine. 2015;**33**(29):3384-3391

[4] Egawa G, Kabashima K. Role of lymphoid structure in skin immunity. Current Topics in Microbiology and Immunology. 2020;**426**:65-82

[5] Kowarsky M, Camunas-Soler J, Kertesz M, et al. Numerous uncharacterized and highly divergent microbes which colonize humans are revealed by circulating cell-free DNA. Proceedings of the National Academy of Sciences of the United States of America. 2017;**114**(36):9623-9628

[6] Aagaard K, Ma J, Antony KM, Ganu R, Petrosino J, Versalovic J. The placenta harbors a unique microbiome. Sci Transl Med. 2014;6(237):237ra65.

[7] Davenport ER, Sanders JG, Song SJ, Amato KR, Clark AG, Knight R. The human microbiome in evolution. BMC Biology. 2017;**15**(1):127

[8] Chen YE, Tsao H. The skin microbiome: Current perspectives and future challenges. Journal of the American Academy of Dermatology. 2013;**69**(1):143-155

[9] Pascal M, Perez-Gordo M, Caballero T, et al. Microbiome and allergic diseases. Frontiers in Immunology. 2018;**9**:1584

[10] Fyhrquist N, Ruokolainen L, Suomalainen A, Lehtimaki S, Veckman V, Vendelin J, et al. Acinetobacter species in the skin microbiota protect against allergic sensitization and inflammation. J Allergy Clin Immunol. 2014; 134(6):1301-1309.e11.

[11] Melli LCFL, Carmo-Rodrigues MS, Araújo-Filho HB, et al. Gut microbiota of children with atopic dermatitis: Controlled study in the metropolitan region of São Paulo, Brazil. Allergol Immunopathol (Madr). 2020;**48**(2):107-115

[12] Pothmann A, Illing T, Wiegand C, Hartmann AA, Elsner P. The microbiome and atopic dermatitis: A review. American Journal of Clinical Dermatology. 2019;**20**(6):749-761

[13] Munera-Campos M, Carrascosa JM. Innovation in atopic dermatitis: From pathogenesis to treatment. Actas Dermo-Sifiliográficas. 2020;**111**(3):205-221

[14] Drislane C, Irvine AD. The role of filaggrin in atopic dermatitis and allergic disease. Annals of Allergy, Asthma & Immunology. 2020;**124**(1):36-43

[15] Bağci IS, Ruzicka T. IL-31: A new key player in dermatology and beyond. The Journal of Allergy and Clinical Immunology 2018;141(3):858-866.

[16] Shin JY, Che DN, Byoung BO, Kang HJ, Kim J, Jang SI. Commiphora myrrha inhibits itch-associated histamine and IL-31 production in stimulated mast cells. Experimental and Therapeutic Medicine. 2019;**18**(3):1914-1920

[17] Newsom M, Bashyam AM, Balogh EA, Feldman SR, Strowd LC. New and emerging systemic treatments for atopic dermatitis. Drugs. 2020;**80**(11):1041-1052

[18] Lowe A, Su J, Tang M, et al. PEBBLES study protocol: A randomised controlled trial to prevent atopic dermatitis, food allergy and sensitisation in infants with a family history of allergic disease using a skin barrier improvement strategy. BMJ Open. 2019;**9**:e024594

[19] Lin T-K, Zhong L, Santiago JL. Anti-inflammatory and skin barrier repair effects of topical application of some plant oils. International Journal of Molecular Sciences. 2018;**19**(1):70

[20] Ornelas J, Routt E, Kallis P, Lev-Tov H. Use of the hCONSORT criteria as a reporting standard for herbal interventions for common dermatoses: A systematic review. The British Journal of Dermatology. 2018;**178**(4):889-896

[21] Dhillon S. Delgocitinib: First approval. Drugs. 2020 Apr;**80**(6):609-615

[22] Newsom M, Bashyam AM, Balogh EA, Feldman SR, Strowd LC. New and emerging systemic treatments for atopic dermatitis. Drugs. 2020;**80**(11):1041-1052

[23] Renert-Yuval Y, Guttman-Yassky E. New treatments for atopic dermatitis targeting beyond IL-4/IL-13 cytokines. Annals of Allergy, Asthma & Immunology. 2020;**124**(1):28-35

[24] Gonzalez T, Biagini-Myers JM, Herr AB, Khurana-Hershey GK. Staphylococcal biofilms in atopic dermatitis. Current Allergy and Asthma Reports. 2017;**17**(12):81

[25] Melanda H. Biofilmes e plantas medicinais: evidência científica. In Master Thesis. Medicinal Plants in Clinical Practice Unity, Celso Pereira. Medicine Faculty. Coimbra University. 2019 (April):1-72.

[26] Myles IA. Allergy as a disease of dysbiosis: Is it time to shift the treatment paradigm? Frontiers in Cellular and Infection Microbiology. 2019;**9**:50

[27] Hendricks AJ, Mills BW, Shi VY. Skin bacterial transplant in atopic dermatitis: Knowns, unknowns and emerging trends. Journal of Dermatological Science. 2019;**95**(2):56-61

[28] Rosignoli C, Thibaut de Menonville S, Orfila D, et al. A topical treatment containing heat-treated lactobacillus johnsonii NCC 533 reduces Staphylococcus aureus adhesion and induces antimicrobial peptide expression in an in vitro reconstructed human epidermis model. Experimental Dermatology. 2018;**27**(4):358-365

[29] Alecsandru D, Valor L, Sánchez-Ramón S, et al. Sublingual therapeutic immunization with a polyvalent bacterial preparation in patients with recurrent respiratory infections: Immunomodulatory effect on antigen-specific memory CD4+ T cells and impact on clinical outcome. Clinical and Experimental Immunology. 2011;**164**(1):100-107

[30] Sánchez-Ramón S, Conejero L, Netea MG, Sancho D, Palomares O, Subiza JL. Trained immunity-based vaccines: A new paradigm for the development of broad-Spectrum anti-infectious formulations. Frontiers in Immunology. 2018;**9**:2936

[31] Kearney SC, Dziekiewicz M, Feleszko W. Immunoregulatory and immunostimulatory responses of bacterial lysates in respiratory infections and asthma. Annals of Allergy, Asthma & Immunology. 2015;**114**(5):364-369

[32] Lau S. Oral application of bacterial lysate in infancy diminishes the prevalence of atopic dermatitis in children at risk for atopy. Benef Microbes. 2014;**5**(2):147-149

[33] Nakatsuji T, Chen TH, Narala S, et al. Antimicrobials from human

skin commensal bacteria protect against Staphylococcus aureus and are deficient in atopic dermatitis. Science Translational Medicine. 2017;**9**:378

[34] Perin B, Addetia A, Qin X. Transfer of skin microbiota between two dissimilar autologous microenvironments: A pilot study. PLoS One. 2019;**14**(12):e0226857

[35] Mashiah J. Efficacy of Fecal Microbial Transplantation Treatment in Adults With Atopic Dermatitis. Tel-Aviv Sourasky Medical Center. 2020. ClinicalTrials.gov Identifier: NCT04283968.

[36] Li Q, Fang H, Dang E, Wang G. The role of ceramides in skin homeostasis and inflammatory skin diseases. Journal of Dermatological Science. 2020;**97**(1):2-8

[37] Nomura T, Wu J, Kabashima K, Guttman-Yassky E. Endophenotypic variations of atopic dermatitis by age, race. and Ethnicity J Allergy Clin Immunol Pract. 2020;**8**(6):1840-1852

Chapter 2

Atopic Dermatitis: From Physiopathology to the Clinics

Ignasi Figueras-Nart and Oscar Palomares-Gracia

Abstract

Atopic dermatitis is a chronic, pruritic, relapsing inflammatory disease with a complex etiopathogenesis. Alterations of the epidermal barrier function together with a predominantly type 2 altered immune response are responsible for the heterogeneous clinical manifestation. Although pruritic eczematous plaques represent the most frequent phenotype, several others are also characteristic. The diagnostic of the disease relies on clinical aspects, and no complimentary tests are needed. In the literature, we can find a significant number of diagnostic and screening biomarkers; however, severity ones are the most reliable and applicable. Patient-tailored treatment is mandatory, as not all the patients equally respond to the same drugs. The newly released therapies, as well as those under investigation, give hope to AD patients.

Keywords: atopic dermatitis, immunology, type 2 immune response, clinical features, eczema, biomarkers, risk factors, treatment, biological agents

1. Introduction

Atopic dermatitis (AD) is a common chronic, pruritic, relapsing, inflammatory systemic disease that affects both children and adults. Patients frequently have high levels of total immunoglobin E (IgE) and a personal or family history of atopic-related diseases.

AD is one of the most common inflammatory cutaneous diseases with an incidence that has tripled in the last 3 decades in industrialized countries. Prevalence in children population is approximately 15–20%, while it is much lower in adults, between 1 and 3%.

Several studies demonstrate that AD has a high impact on patients' quality of life (QoL). For some of them, the impairment in QoL is more significant than in some other chronic diseases such as hypertension, diabetes, or even psoriasis [1].

In this chapter, we will make a dual approach to AD. First, we will concentrate on the immunological mechanisms of AD and then will discuss the clinical and therapeutic aspects of the disease.

2. Immunological mechanisms of AD

2.1 Immunological mechanisms underlying atopic dermatitis

The immune system is a very complex and interactive network of cells and molecules to protect the host against potentially dangerous pathogens while keeping at the same time a state of tolerance against self and innocuous non-self-antigens [2, 3]. The immune system employs a large number of molecular and cellular mechanisms that must be tightly regulated to perform this vital function. Alterations on these mechanisms lead to the appearance of immune-related diseases such as recurrent infections, autoimmunity, tumor tolerance, organ rejection, as well as allergic and skin diseases such as AD [2, 4–6].

AD is one of the most prevalent chronic inflammatory diseases of the skin affecting both children and adults [7, 8]. The clinical features that characterize the disease are dry and scaly skin, eczema lesions, and chronic itching. AD is a very complex and debilitating disease that should be considered as a systemic disease associated with different comorbidities. The development of AD depends on the integration of multiple factors such as genetic background, environmental exposure, skin barrier, and immune alterations [9–11]. All these factors cooperate and synergize leading to the clinical manifestations of AD. Over the last years, our understanding on the immunological mechanisms underlying AD has significantly improved [12]. Today, it is well accepted that the inflammatory component of AD is mainly driven by aberrant type 2 immune responses, which significantly contribute also to barrier defects and itching [5, 13]. Other immune responses including Th17, Th22, and, to a lesser extent, Th1 cells can also contribute to AD at different stages of the disease as well as in different subsets of patients and phenotypes [11, 14, 15].

2.2 Orchestration of type 2 immune responses

The immune system employs type 2 immune responses to combat parasites and helminths, as well as toxins and venoms [16, 17]. Parasites are pathogens very large in size that cannot be engulfed and eliminated by innate immune cells, and dangerous venoms/toxins might rapidly spread throughout the body. Therefore, the main aim of type 2 immune responses is to expulse away the pathogen from the body or destroy the toxins, thus avoiding their systemic dissemination and the lethal consequences for the host. Aberrant type 2 immune responses, due to different and sometimes unknown etiologies, might lead to the development of allergic diseases such as asthma or food allergy as well as to skin diseases such as AD [2, 4, 18]. Initially, AD was regarded as a Th2-mediated disease; however, recent findings showed that type 2 innate lymphoid cells (ILC2s) and other innate immune and effector cells also contribute to the orchestration of these responses. Therefore, the term type 2-mediate disease is more adequate according to our current knowledge [19, 20].

Different cell subsets from both arms of the immune system, as well as tissues and non-hematopoietic cells, directly contribute to the orchestration of type 2 immune responses, both locally and systemically [19]. Under normal conditions, the presence of helminths or toxic substances triggers the production of large amounts of alarmins such as TSLP, IL-33, or IL-25 by epithelial cells (ECs). Alarmins directly activate and expand ILC2s by mechanisms depending on IL-7 and condition the capacity of dendritic cells (DCs) to induce T helper (Th)2 and type 2 CD8+ cytotoxic T-cell (Tc2) responses by mechanisms depending on IL-4 [21]. Activated ILC2s, Th2, and Tc2 cells produce type 2 cytokines such as IL-4, IL-13, or IL-5, which contribute to the recruitment and activation of different effector cells such as eosinophils, basophils, and mast cells to the inflamed tissue. Type 2 cytokines also participate in the activation of non-hematopoietic cells and tissues, which in cooperation with the activated immune effectors' cells aim at eliminating the potentially dangerous invading pathogen/toxin, avoiding systemic dissemination.

2.3 Dendritic cells connect innate and adaptive immune responses

DCs are antigen professional presenting cells (APCs) that link innate and adaptive immune responses [2, 22]. They are localized in all peripheral tissues, circulating in the blood and lymphoid organs. Their primary function is to scan and collect antigens in the periphery (skin, airways, or gut), process these antigens into peptide fragments, and present them in the context of MHC molecules to naïve T cells. DCs express costimulatory molecules and produce polarizing cytokines, which, together with their migratory capacity, empower them as the essential APCs in the priming of T cell responses [15, 23].

Depending on the type of encountered antigen and the signals that DCs receive in the periphery and during the travel to the lymph node, they can generate different types of effector CD4+ T cells [24, 25]. When DCs encounter intracellular pathogens (viruses or bacteria), they produce large amounts of IL-12 and induce IFN-γ-producing Th1 cells that in turn activate NK cells and CD8+ T cells to combat these infections. Aberrant Th1 responses also associate other autoimmune diseases [25]. In contrast, extracellular pathogens (bacteria or fungi) condition DCs to produce large quantities of IL-23, IL-1β, TGF-β, and IL-6, thus promoting the generation of IL-17A-producing Th17 cells that contribute to neutrophilic infiltration to eliminate these pathogens. Alterations of Th17 responses have been associated with different autoimmune diseases and psoriasis [26]. Under certain circumstances, mucosal DCs can also generate IL-9-producing Th9 or IL-22-producing Th22 cells, which contribute to activate mast cells and to promote epidermal hyperplasia, respectively [24, 26]. As above discussed, the presence of parasites or venoms activates ECs and instructs DCs to polarize Th2 cells producing large amounts of type 2 cytokines such as IL-4, IL-13, IL-5, or IL-9. Aberrant Th2 responses are the main drivers of allergic diseases and AD [12, 25]. In addition to these effectors CD4+ T-cell responses, DCs can also generate regulatory T cells with potent suppressive capacity, which play a crucial role in keeping homeostasis avoiding excessive immune activation and tolerance induction [2, 3, 18, 27].

In humans, blood DCs are classified into two main groups: (i) myeloid dendritic cells (mDCs) and (ii) plasmacytoid dendritic cells (pDCs) [28]. According to the expression of specific markers, mDCs can be further divided into type 1 mDCs and type 2 mDCs [28–30].

pDCs are the primary producers of type I IFNs and are essential in antiviral responses, whereas different subsets of mDCs contribute to the orchestration of different types of immune responses. Both mDCs and pDCs are different phenotypic and functional DC subsets that cooperate to integrate and mount immune responses.

In the healthy skin, under non-inflammatory conditions, the number of DCs is relatively low with a clear predominance of epidermal and dermal Langerhans cells (LCs) [12, 31]. In contrast, the number and composition of DC subsets in the lesional skin of AD patients are altered with significant infiltration of inflammatory dendritic epidermal and dermal cells (IDECs and IDDCs, respectively) [12, 31]. DCs in the skin of AD patients express high levels of the high-affinity receptor for IgE (FcεRI), which might play a critical role in the priming and expansion of memory T cells. Besides, after IgE-FcεRI cross-linking, DCs produce a plethora of chemokines that add to the recruitment of Th2 cells and other inflammatory cells into the skin, thus enhancing inflammation. IDECs can also migrate to lymph node and polarize and increase the frequency of Th2 cells but also Th1, Th17, and Th22 as observed during the most chronic phases of AD [12, 31]. Overall, DCs play an essential role in the initiation and maintenance of type 2 immune responses in the context of AD as well as in the generation of other Th cell subsets detected during the chronic phases and in different phenotypes of AD patients.

2.4 The immunopathogenesis of AD

The knowledge of the immunological mechanisms involved in the pathogenesis of AD has significantly improved over the last years. There are three phases in AD development involving different cytokines and cellular signatures that account for the clinical manifestations of the disease: (i) initial non-lesional stage, (ii) acute stage, and (iii) chronic stage.

2.4.1 Initial non-lesional stage

The structural integrity and permeability to environmental insults are severely compromised in susceptible patients displaying skin barrier defects [5, 10]. These skin alterations might be originated due to different factors including genetic susceptibility (mutations in filaggrin and/or other key genes for stratum corneum and skin integrity), alterations in tight junction proteins (TJ), dysregulation of skin lipid composition, changes in pH, altered microbiome, high transepithelial water loss (TWEL), or high susceptibility to infections and irritants. These skin barrier defects allow the penetration of large amounts of allergens, pathogen-derived antigens, and/or other environmental insults into the lower epidermal layers, leading to the activation of keratinocytes [7]. Skin DCs uptake the encountered allergens and migrate to the closer lymph nodes conditioned by keratinocyte-derived alarmins such as TSLP, IL-33, or IL-25. These alarmins also activate tissue-resident ILC2s, which produce large amounts of type 2 cytokines facilitating DC migration and recruitment of inflammatory cells into the skin [7, 10]. Under these circumstances, DCs polarize naïve CD4+ T cells into allergen-specific Th2 cells by mechanisms depending on IL-4. The clonal expansion and activation of Th2 cells significantly contribute to IgE class-switching at the B level. The generated IgE+ B cells differentiate into plasma cells that produce large amounts of allergen-specific IgE antibodies that bind to the surface of mast cells and basophils, leading to the allergic sensitization [2, 4]. The induced Th2 cells home back and infiltrate the skin through lymph and circulation, leading to the classical skin inflammation observed of this initial stage even in the absence of skin lesions.

2.4.2 Acute stage

During the acute stage of AD, activated Th2 cells and ILC2s produce large amounts of IL-4, IL-13, IL-31, and IL-5 [12, 24]. IL-5 favors eosinophil recruitment into the skin and IL-31 in cooperation with IL-4 and IL-13 play a critical role in itching, thus initiating the vicious circle of itching-scratching that contributes to increase the damage of the already altered skin barrier and to enhance inflammation [12]. IL-31 directly act on sensory neurons, but it also promotes the growth of sensory nerves and skin hyperinnervation [32, 33]. IL-4 not only contributes to increasing the expression of IL-31 [34] but also together with IL-13 to sensitize neurons to a large variety of pruritogens such IL-33 and TSLP that increase after scratching, thus potentially contributing to chronic itch [32]. IL-4 and IL-13 also directly act on keratinocytes by inhibiting their differentiation, the production of antimicrobial peptides (AMPs), and altering lipid metabolism, thus enhancing barrier disruption. Six IL-13-activated keratinocytes produce an extensive battery of chemokines such as CCL17 (TARC), CCL26 (eotaxin), CCL18, and CCL22. In cooperation with the increment of vascular permeability induced by IL-4 through the increased of vascular cell adhesion molecule-1 (VCAM-1) on vascular endothelial cells, a massive infiltration of different types of inflammatory cells and vascular leakage takes place [5, 7]. Collectively, all these mechanisms account for the typical clinical symptoms of the AD acute stage, including itching and eczema lesions characterized by edema and spongiosis.

2.4.3 Chronic stage

The perpetuation of this predominant type 2 inflammation might lead to the chronicity of the disease [5]. In this phase, inflammation increases and persists due to constant activation of keratinocytes, vascular endothelium, inflammatory cells, and chronic itching. Remarkably, in the chronic stage, other Th cell subsets including IFN-γ-producing Th1, IL-17-producing Th17, and IL-22-producing Th22 are also infiltrating the skin lesions [11, 15]. Depending on the AD subtypes, the relative frequency and contribution of these inflammatory Th cell subsets might vary significantly [11, 35, 36]. For example, in Asian AD patients as well as in some AD children subtypes, IL-17-producing Th17 cells might contribute to parakeratosis resembling typical features of psoriasis. In European-American, African American, and children AD patients, IL-22 produced by Th22 cells in cooperation with high levels of type 2 cytokines IL-4/IL-13 reinforce defective barrier function. It also enhances keratinocyte proliferation and promotes epidermal hyperplasia, leading to the lichenification and chronic itching typical of chronic stage [5, 10, 11, 35, 36].

3. Clinical features of AD

Although AD frequently appears during childhood and tends to subside as the patient grows, there is a considerable number of patients who persist in adulthood.

Recently, adult-onset and elderly onset phenotypes have been described [37, 38].

The essential features of AD are eczematous lesions and pruritus. Former can be acute, subacute, or chronic.

The clinical presentations, the lesion type and its distribution, are age specific, and this is a crucial aspect to consider when examining patients so as not to miss diagnose them.

AD phenotypes can be stratified according to multiple characteristics. One of the most used is the age-related clinical stratification, which classifies patients into four groups [39].

Infantile AD: Patients from 0 to 2 years present with an acute form of eczema, which typically affects cheeks, face, sparing nasal-labial triangle, scalp, trunk, and extensor surfaces of the limbs. The napkin area is typically respected.

Children AD: From 2 to puberty patients show subacute-to-chronic eczema that affects the flexural folds, dorsal aspects of the limbs, perioral area, and napkin area.

Adult AD: Adults typically present with a chronic or lichenified (**Figure 1**) and symmetric eczema that involves flexures, wrist, ankles, eyelids, and cheeks. In patients with a longstanding AD, a selective involvement of the neck and dorsal aspect of the hands is frequent, showing lichenified brown lesions that resemble dirt (**Figure 2**).

Elderly AD: AD in elderly presents with widespread chronic eczematous lesions with significant itch (**Figure 3**). It is usually misdiagnosed as cutaneous T-cell lymphoma, allergic contact dermatitis, or other types of eczema. Further information is needed regarding the exact clinical presentation so as not to underestimate its real prevalence.

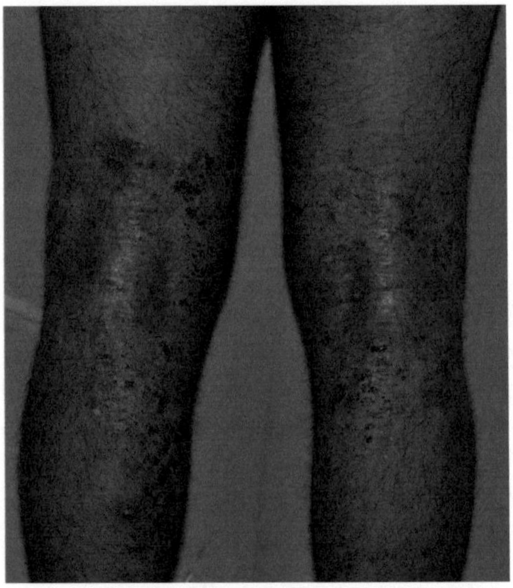

Figure 1.
Lichenified lesions on the posterior part of the legs.

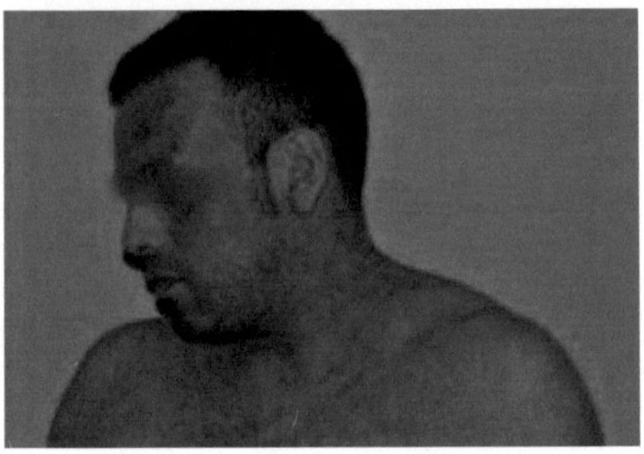

Figure 2.
Chronic eczema in an adult patient with lichenified brown lesions on the lateral aspects of the neck that resemble dirt.

Patients can also be classified according to the age of onset [39]. Bieber et al. proposed six phenotypes, which included very early-onset (3 months–2 years), early-onset (2–6 yeas), childhood-onset (6–14 years), adolescent-onset (14–20 years), adult-onset (20–60 years), and very late-onset (>60 years). The majority of patients fall into the first group; however, adult-onset is a recently identified group, which represents about 20% of all the cases. The latter group includes two subsets, those with AD in the past and a long period of remission and those with a very late-onset.

It is important to consider that patients can present not only with widespread lesions but also with localized or morphologically distinct phenotypes.

Localized variants include selective eczema of the nipples, hands, eyelids, periauricular area, cheilitis, subnasal region, and genital area. The head and neck type are typical of the adult group and show involvement of the upper trunk and scalp.

Morphological variants comprise the follicular type, which presents as aggregated follicular papules, the papulo-lichenoid variant, the prurigo variant that resembles a prurigo nodularis, the nummular variant, and erythroderma [5, 37, 40] (**Figure 4**).

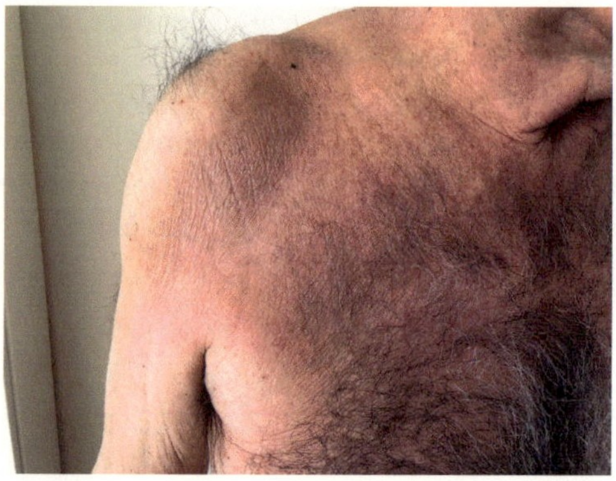

Figure 3.
Widespread eczema in an elderly patient.

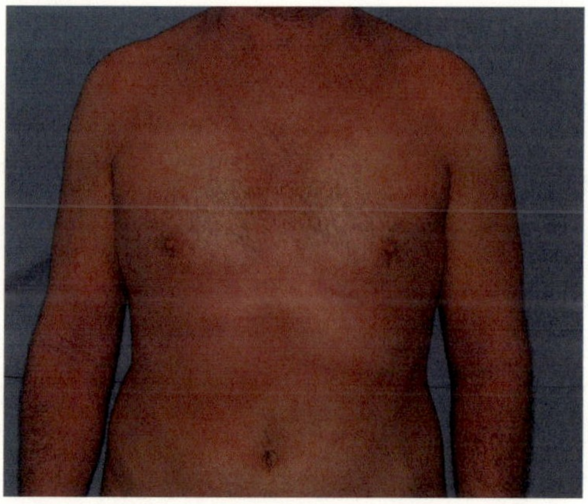

Figure 4.
Erythrodermic variant of AD.

Silvestre Salvador et al. [37] recently described and classified the clinical forms of presentation of AD in adult patients. They identified 11 groups: lichenified/exudative flexural dermatitis, head-and-neck eczema, seborrheic dermatitis-like dermatitis, portrait dermatitis, hand eczema, generalized eczema, prurigo nodularis, nummular eczema, erythroderma, psoriasiform dermatitis, and multiple lesions of lichen simplex.

3.1 Diagnostic of AD

The diagnostic of AD is based on clinical features since no specific biomarkers or histological hallmarks exist. It relies on the morphology and distribution of the lesions, clinical history, and other clinical signs.

Multiple sets of diagnostic criteria have been developed since 1980 when Hanifin-Rajka proposed the first, which included major and minor features. It requires 3 out of the four major and 3 out of the 23 minor criteria to establish a diagnosis. Later, the "United Kingdom Working Party" settled a set, which followed the essence of the Hanifin-Rajka's, but adapted it for epidemiological and clinical studies [5].

In 2003, Eichenfield et al. [41] revised the original criteria and elaborated a set dividing features into essential, important, and associated (**Table 1**). It also includes exclusionary criteria to help with the differential diagnostic. Probably, these criteria are the most used in a clinical setting.

In 2016, Liu P et al. [42] proposed an easy-to-use set for adolescents and adults. They based the diagnostic on the presence of symmetric eczema for more than 6 months associated to one or more of the following: family or personal history of atopic-related diseases, eosinophilia, and elevated total or specific IgE.

Diagnostic criteria for SD			
Essential features (must be present)	Pruritus		
	Eczema (acute, subacute or chronic)	Typical morphology and age-specific patterns	Facial, neck, and extensor involvement in infants and children
			Current or prior flexural lesions in any age group
			Sparing of groin and axillary regions
		Chronic or relapsing	
Important features (seen in most of the cases, adding support to the diagnosis)	Early onset		
	Atopy	Personal and/or family history	
		IgE reactivity	
	Xerosis		
Associated features (help to suggest the diagnosis of AD but are too non-specific to be used for defining or detecting AD)	Atypical vascular response		
	Keratosis pilaris/pityriasis alba/hyperlinear palms/ichthyosis		
	Ocular or periorbital changes		
	Other regional findings		
	Perifollicular accentuation/lichenification/prurigo lesions		
Exclusionary conditions	Scabies		
	Seborrheic dermatitis		
	Contact dermatitis		
	Ichthyosis		
	Cutaneous T-cell lymphoma		
	Psoriasis		
	Photosensitivity dermatoses		
	Immune deficiency diseases		
	Erythroderma of other causes		

Adapted from Eichenfield et al. [41].

Table 1.
Diagnostic criteria proposed by Eichenfield et al. in 2003.

3.2 Approach to the patient with AD

When considering the diagnostic of AD, it is crucial making a thorough clinical history, which includes information regarding the chronicity of eczema, the presence of itch, and the personal and family history of atopy. In children, AD is one of the first diagnostics to consider, while in the adult population, probably due to a lack of familiarity with adult-onset disease and even when dealing with patients with a compatible clinical picture, the first diagnostic suspicion tends to be contact dermatitis. Physical examination is also mandatory to determine the morphology and distribution of the lesions, which can help to consider or even establish the diagnostic [37].

There are controversies regarding complementary tests, which are useful at ruling out differential diagnostics. According to the AAD guidelines, AD is a diagnostic of exclusion and should only be established after excluding other diseases [43].

Patch testing should be considered in patients with adult-onset disease, those with a chronic disease who fail to respond to adequate treatment, patients with atypical or changing distribution, as well as patients with patterns suggestive of allergic contact dermatitis. Patch test should always be assessed according to clinical history to determine the relevance of the results [37].

The utility of the prick test is somewhat controversial. A prick for airborne allergens could be useful in adults with an airborne pattern eczema involving the face, particularly eyelid area, neck, and exposed regions of upper limbs. Testing for food allergies might be of help in pediatric patients with generalized eczema that worsen when exposed to certain foods, but also in adult patients who are sensitized to pollen, as pollen-related foods can cause cross-reaction with airborne allergens and trigger flares. Ruling out a protein contact dermatitis could be indicated in patients with chronic hand eczema that flares when handling food [37, 44].

A blood test is not mandatory but can be useful at supporting the diagnostic of AD. High IgE levels and eosinophilia are frequent in these patients. Other parameters such as lactate dehydrogenase (LDH), serum thymic activation regulator chemokine (sTARC)/CCL17, CCL27, cationic eosinophilic protein (CEP), and antitransglutaminase antibodies may provide with information regarding the severity or helping in the differential diagnostic (see biomarkers).

Although the histopathologic picture of atopic dermatitis does not differ from other types of eczema, a skin biopsy may help rule out other diagnostics such as cutaneous T-cell lymphoma (CTCL), psoriasis, or drug reactions [37].

Including a simple blood test with hemogram, liver function, renal function, LDH, total IgE (and specific if the clinical history suggests it), IgA, and antitransglutaminase antibodies would be reasonable during the initial diagnostic workup. Indications for a patch test and prick test are those specified before.

3.3 Assessment of the disease severity and impact on the quality of life

After setting up the diagnostic of AD, it is essential to assess the severity of the disease and its impact on patient's quality of life.

3.3.1 Severity

Several scales evaluate the severity; some of them include just objective signs, while others also include subjective patient's symptoms.

Most of the scales are composite score systems, which assess different aspects of the disease (**Table 2**).

Severity				**Quality of life**			
Scale	**Score**	**Description**	**Msc**	**Scale**	**Score**	**Description**	**Msc**
SCORAD	0–103	<25 mild 25–50 moderate >50 severe	8.7	HADS	0–42 (A/D)	0–7 normal 8–10 borderline abnormal 11–21 abnormal	N/A
EASI	0–72	≤7 mild >7–21 moderate >21 severe	6.6	DLQI	0–30	0–1 no effect at all on patient's life 2–5 small effect 6–10 moderate effect 11–20 very large effect 21–30 extremely large effect	4
IGA	0–4	0 clear 1 almost clear 2 mild 3 moderate 4 severe	N/A				
			Symptoms				
POEM	0–28	0–2 clear or almost clear 3–7 mild 8–16 moderate 17–24 severe 25–28 very severe					3.4
VAS pruritus	0–10	The higher the score, the more severe the pruritus					2–3
VAS sleep	0–10	The higher the score, the more sleeplessness					2–3

SCORAD, scoring of atopic dermatitis; EASI, eczema area and severity index; HADS, hospital anxiety and depression scale; DLQI, dermatology life quality index; POEM, patient-oriented eczema measures for eczema; VAS, visual analogue scale; MSC, minimal significant change.

Table 2.
Scales of severity and quality of life.

The most used in European countries is the Scoring of Atopic Dermatitis (SCORAD). It first evaluates the body surface area (BSA) affected and then gives a score from 0 to 3 for each of the following clinical features: erythema, edema, excoriation, swelling/crusts, lichenification, and xerosis. Finally, the patient is asked to rank pruritus and sleeplessness from 0 (best situation) to 10 (worst situation), giving a total score that ranges from 0 to 103, being the latter the most severe. It is considered a score from 0 to 25 as a mild disease, 25–50 as moderate, and 50 and above as severe.

Eczema area and severity index (EASI) is a scale based on PASI score.

EASI is a more objective tool, which does not include the patient's symptoms, which is widely used in the US and also in the setting of most of the clinical trials. It divides the body into four parts, head and neck, trunk, upper limbs, and lower limbs. The first step is to assess the affected surface in each of the zones and then score erythema, edema, excoriation, and lichenification from 0 to 3. Each score is multiplied by a specific quotient, obtaining a final number that ranges from 0 to 72.

The patient-oriented eczema measures for eczema (POEM) is a symptom score that measures the subjective symptoms of the patient. The final result ranges from 0 to 28, being the latter the worst.

Investigator global assessment (IGA) is an easy-to-use scale that describes the overall appearance of the lesions and scores the severity from 0 to 3, 0 means a clear, 1 almost clear, 2 mild, 3 moderate, and 4 severe disease. Unlike the other three scales, it is not a validated score, but a global assessment of the disease.

3.3.2 Quality of life

Assessing disease impact on patient's quality of life is as important as evaluating the severity.

There are over ten disease-specific tests available for AD and more than 25 generic instruments that can be used in AD [45]. Each of these tools focuses on different aspects of the disease, not only regarding the patient but also their family or close relatives. **Table 2** shows two of the most used scales in assessing QoL.

There are also non-disease-specific questionnaires that study the school or work productivity, focusing not only on work absenteeism but also on presenteeism. One of the most known is WPAI (Work Productivity and Activity Impairment), which is composed of 6 questions regarding the effect of the disease on the ability to work and perform regular activities.

3.4 Biomarkers in AD

Biomarkers are an interesting matter of debate nowadays. Although there is plenty of literature on the topic, the utility and applicability of them still present some concerns.

A biomarker is a common term used across the atopic dermatitis literature. There are two definitions proposed by the World Health Organization (WHO) and by the National Institutes of Health (NIH) biomarkers definition group, which largely overlap. The WHO defines it as "any substance, structure or process that can be measured in the body or its products and influence or predict the incidence of outcome or disease. Biomarkers can be classified into markers of exposure, effect and susceptibility" [46], while the NIH definition is "a characteristic that is objectively measured and evaluated as an indicator of normal biological processes, pathogenic processes, or pharmacologic responses to a therapeutic intervention." [47].

There are two types of biomarkers, those used for selection or stratification of the patients and those used for monitoring the clinical response.

The former includes screening, diagnostic, prognostic, and predictive biomarkers, while the latter comprises severity and pharmacodynamic markers [48].

Screening biomarkers: Several biomarkers could help in the screening. Mutations in the filaggrin gene are present in up to 30% of the AD patients. R501X and 2282del4 are the most frequent and are dose dependent. These may predict a higher risk of eczema herpeticum and an earlier onset of the disease [49, 50].

Other parameters, such as high levels of cord IgE, infantile a-lymphotoxin and FcεRI-β during pregnancy, as well as high TEWL and SPINK5/LEKTI, could also be useful as screening biomarkers [48].

Diagnostic biomarkers: Although the AD diagnostic is clinical, some biomarkers could help to decant the balance toward AD. Total serum IgE is a useful parameter for dividing patients into intrinsic and extrinsic phenotypes. Up to 20% of patients belong to the intrinsic group, with normal levels of IgE. Consequently, it is an unreliable biomarker for diagnostic purposes.

Filaggrin and leukotriene B4 serum levels could be two valuable biomarkers, as they have been shown to differ from healthy controls significantly. AD patients tend to present higher levels of the former and lower of the latter [51].

Prognostic biomarkers: The purpose of these markers is to estimate the course and evolution of the disease. The only known parameter in this group is the presence of some mutations in the filaggrin gene, which could determine a more severe course of the disease [48].

Predictive biomarkers: This group identifies patients that are most likely to respond to a specific therapy. Currently, as new targeted therapies are arising, there is an evident lack of such biomarkers that help to classify and assign a given treatment.

Recently, Wollenberg et al. described that higher levels of serum periostin and dipeptidyl-dipeptidase 4 (DDP4) conditioned a better response to anti-IL-13 therapies. On the other hand, the presence of single-nucleotide polymorphism (SNP) in the gene promoter region of UGT1A9 is related to low mycophenolate blood levels, and thus a worse response to the drug. Increasing the dose could solve this lack of response [48, 52].

Pharmacodynamic biomarkers: These biomarkers might be relevant when planning therapeutic regimens for AD patients. Although scarcely used, these may help to personalize and enhance efficiently of some systemic treatments.

Tacrolimus is metabolized by CYP3A4 and CYP3A5. CYP3A4*22 and CYP3A5*3 are seen in slow metabolizers, leading to high blood levels. CYP3A5*3 is associated with a fast metabolism, and it entails low blood levels.

Increased activity of UGT1A9 caused by SNPs can lead to a lack of response to mycophenolate due to low blood levels [48].

Azathioprine (AZA) adverse events can be predicted by genotyping thiopurine methyltransferase. The risk of myelotoxicity and liver toxicity can be assessed by monitoring AZA metabolites 6-thioguanine nucleotides and 6-methylmercaptopurine ribonucleotides [53].

Severity biomarkers: Most of the known biomarkers belong to this group. It is essential to distinguish between those biomarkers studied in longitudinal studies, which give information of the evolution of the parameter along the time and in response to the treatment and those derived from cross-sectional studies, which provide with an objective measure of severity at a given moment. Lately, most of the efforts on biomarkers are focused on identifying combinations of biomarkers, which better predict the severity of the disease [54]. Thijs et al. proposed two panels of biomarkers, the first of them [55] is made up of TARC, PARC, IL-22, and sIL-2R and correlates much better with the disease severity than each of the biomarkers alone. The same group elaborated a second panel composed of TARC, IL-22, and sIL-2R, which allowed to predict EASI with a sensitivity of 100% and specificity of 88.9% [56].

Table 3 summarizes these biomarkers.

3.5 Risk factors

Several factors have been associated with the development of AD. Some are regarded as risk factors, while others have a protective role.

Atopy family history and loss-of-function mutations in the gene of filaggrin are two clear risk factors for AD. About 70% of the patients have a positive family history of atopic diseases. The OR for children with one parent affected, compared to those without any, is 2–3, while those with the two parents affected it is 3–5.

FLG-null mutations condition a more severe, persistent and early-onset disease with a higher tendency to eczema herpeticum [43, 60].

Kelleher et al., have recently described that skin barrier dysfunction at 2 days and 2 months of life, as well as neonatal adiposity, increases the risk of AT during the first year of life.

Biomarker	Cross-sectional studies	Longitudinal studies	Conclusion
sTARC/CCL17	Yes	Yes	Potential biomarker for severity and evolution of the disease. Best characterized biomarker [54]
Total IgE	Yes	Yes	Could be a good biomarker for the severity but not for the disease evolution [54]
cTACK/CCL27	Yes	No	Potential biomarker for severity [54]
ECP	Yes	Yes	Questionable value as a severity and evolution biomarker [54]
EDN	Yes	No	Potential biomarker for the severity. Could be a predictor of relapse in severe AD [57]
LDH	Yes	No	Potential biomarker for severity [54]
Periostin	Yes	No	Good correlation with disease severity and chronicity [58]
IL-18	Yes	No	Potential biomarker for severity [54]
E-selectin	Yes	No	Potential biomarker for severity [54]
CD30	Yes	No	Potential biomarker for severity [54]
IL-2R, IL-4R, IL-31, and tryptase	Yes	No	May correlate with severity. More studies needed [54, 59]

ECP, eosinophil cationic protein; EDN, eosinophil derived neurotoxin; LDH, lactate dehydrogenase.

Table 3.
Severity biomarkers.

An increase in the transepidermal water loss (TWEL) at 2 days and 2 months of life conditions to a higher incidence of AD at 6 and 12 months, regardless of the FLG mutations, family history, or presence of itchy flexural rash at 2 months [61].

Besides, a fat mass of the 80th percentile or higher at day two might also be a predictor for AD at 6 and 12 months of age [62].

Risk and protective factors are summarized in **Table 4**.

3.6 Comorbidities

Compared to non-AD patients, patients with AD have a higher incidence of comorbidities that include not only the atopic march associated diseases but also other disorders. The sequential appearance, since early ages, of atopic dermatitis, allergic rhinitis, asthma, and rhinitis is known as the atopic march and is frequently seen together in patients with AD. Other diseases as chronic pulmonary disease, chronic rhinosinusitis, urticaria, autoimmune disorders, conjunctivitis, eosinophilic esophagitis, nasal polyposis, obesity, bacterial, fungal, and viral infections are also seen more frequently in these patients. Neuropsychiatric disorders including anxiety, depression, attention deficit hyperactivity disorder (ADHD), and sleep disturbances are also more prevalent in AD patients than controls.

In a study from the US, authors showed that not only these diseases are more frequent among AD patients but also that are more likely to occur in those with severe disease compared to less severe patients [64].

Finally, an increase in cardiovascular events has been reported in these patients. Andersen et al. showed that this higher incidence was due to an increased burden of comorbidities and detrimental lifestyle behavior [65]. Brunner et al., later suggested

Risk factors	• Family history • Loss-of-function mutations in FLG gene • Parents educations: higher education–higher risk • Urban zones • Domestic animals: cat increases the risk • Indoor exposition to chemicals • Environmental tobacco smoke • Traffic exhaust
Not risk factors	• Age at which food is introduced • Socioeconomical status • Type of delivery • Birth weight
Protective factors	• Hydrolyzed formulas or exposition to probiotics • Exposition to endotoxin, dogs and farm animals at early ages • Unpasteurized milk • Helminthic infections

Table 4.
Risk and protective factors for developing AD [43, 60, 63].

that inflammatory mediators involved in the atherosclerosis development such as CCL7, IL16, PI3, and E-selectin would be responsible for this increase in the incidence and that they were strongly related to the severity of cutaneous inflammation rather than obesity or lifestyle behavior [66].

4. Treatment

There is not a single approach to the treatment of patients with AD. It is a patient-tailored treatment, which depends on the patients' predominant symptoms and past medical history.

The therapy aims to control the skin barrier disruption, the altered immune response, and microbial infections, as well as pruritus [67].

4.1 Topical treatment

Baseline treatment for AD is moisturizers to help to prevent water loss and maintaining skin hydration. Emollients, humectants, or occlusive agents should be used as a maintenance treatment for all patients with AD. The recommended weekly amount is 250-500 g in adult patients and about 100 g in children.

The use of emollients in inflamed skin is poorly tolerated, it is advised to treat the inflammation first with topical treatments and then apply the moisturizer, at least twice a day [68].

According to the European guidelines for the treatment of AD, an "emollient" is a "topical formulation with vehicle-type substances lacking active ingredients," whereas "emollients plus" refers to "topical formulations with vehicle-type substances and additional active, non-medicated substances" and are meant to target specific lesions [68].

Simpson et al. showed that strict emollient therapy from birth in children at a high risk of developing AD (a parent or full sibling with AD, asthma, or allergic rhinitis) was a practical preventive approach [69].

It is also essential to keep optimal skin hygiene. There are some controversies regarding daily bath; however, a short bath of up to 5 minutes with bath oils or non-irritant and low-allergen formulas, to eliminate crusts and bacterial contaminants, is advised.

Adding antiseptics to the bathwater may be useful in cases that show bacterial superinfection [68].

4.2 Topical anti-inflammatory treatment and phototherapy

Topical corticosteroids and calcineurin inhibitors are the treatments of choice for flares in patients with mild disease (SCORAD <25/EASI <7). Moderate or recurrent cases (SCORAD 25–50/EASI 7–21) require proactive therapy with more potent corticosteroids, calcineurin inhibitors, or phototherapy. The proactive scheme consists of daily application of emollients to unaffected skin combined with intermittent use (twice weekly) of the anti-inflammatory drug in usually affected sites. Studies have proven long-term security and efficacy in reducing relapses [68].

The amount of topical anti-inflammatory drugs should follow the fingertip unit rule (0.5 g), which is the adequate amount for application to two adult palm area (approx. 2% of adult body surface area).

Phototherapy, UVA1 and narrow-band UVB, has shown its long-term efficacy in AD in multiple studies. Except for high doses of UVA1, it is not indicated during flares, but in pruritic and lichenified chronic forms. Most of the times, concomitant use of emollients and/or anti-inflammatory therapy is advised.

Severe patients (SCORAD > 50/EASI > 20) require a more aggressive approach with immunosuppressive agents or biologicals.

Crisaborole is a topical phosphodiesterase 4 (PDE4) blocker approved in the US for the treatment of mild-to-moderate AD in patients 2 years old and older, which has shown to be more effective than the vehicle alone. There are no comparative studies with topical corticosteroids or calcineurin inhibitors [67, 68, 70].

Topical Janus kinase inhibitors are still not licensed for the treatment of AD, but they are in the pipeline of multiple laboratories that are currently conducting phase II studies.

4.3 Systemic treatment

Antihistamines: Although the use of systemic antihistamines is widespread in the treatment of pruritus in AD patients, the scarce studies available have shown a minimal effect on decreasing pruritus. First-generation anti-H1 have a sedative effect that can help in decreasing nocturnal itch, but with impaired sleep quality.

Although there is not enough evidence to support the use of both first and second-generation anti-H1, the former should be used with caution in patients with AD and sleep disturbances.

Corticosteroids: Systemic corticosteroids have been widely used for the treatment of AD. Both European and American guidelines recommend to use them for short periods (up to 7–10 days), for treating acute flares, at a daily dose of 0.5 mg/kg. Long-term use is discouraged due to side effects. A possible rebound after withdrawal should be considered when treating these patients [71].

Immunosuppressive agents: These are the drugs of choice for most of the moderate-to-severe patients. Cyclosporine A (CsA) is the only approved systemic drug for the treatment of AD in Europe. It has shown its efficacy both in adults and children, although it is not approved under 18 years old. CsA is indicated in chronic, severe cases of AD for a maximum of 2 years in a row. Is a fast-acting drug with an onset of the efficacy within the first 2 months, but it has a rapid relapse once stopped. The most used doses range from 2.5 to 5 mg/kg/day. There is no clear consensus on how to start, some authors opt for starting at low doses (2.5 mg/kg/day) and increase the dose 0.5 mg/kg/day every 2–4 weeks depending on the clinical response, up to a maximum of 5 mg/kg/day. Some others prefer starting at high doses and reduce the dose until the minimum efficacious dose. The main concerns regarding the use of this therapy are toxicities and interactions. Nephrotoxicity is the main side effect, which is more likely to occur in doses over 5 mg/kg/day, elderly patients and previous renal impairment. Patients under treatment with CsA are advised to take blood pressure regularly and monitor for renal parameters [71].

Other immunosuppressants such as methotrexate (15–25 mg/week), azathioprine (1–3 mg/kg/day), and mycophenolate mofetil (up to 3 g/day) are used off-label. These tend to have a slower onset of the effect, around 8–12 weeks, but with a more prolonged residual effect once the treatment is stopped [71].

No studies are comparing the efficacy of the three agents; however, Eckert et al. have recently shown that patients receiving mycophenolate mofetil required more oral corticosteroid than the other treatments, whereas those receiving CsA were the patients who needed the least [72].

Two studies compared the overall efficacy of methotrexate and azathioprine and concluded to be equivalent [73, 74].

It is essential to regularly monitor these patients for possible side effects, mainly liver toxicity.

Biological agents: Despite all the immunosuppressive armamentarium, some patients still show a lack of efficacy. Biologicals are highly effective therapies with an immunomodulatory effect that specifically target inflammatory cells or mediators. Most of the biologicals developed or in development for AD target cytokines of the T2 response.

Dupilumab is the first biological licensed for AD. It is a fully human monoclonal antibody that blocks a chain of the IL-4 receptor, which is common in the receptor for IL-4 and IL-13. It is approved as first-line therapy for adult moderate-to-severe AD who are candidates to systemic therapy. Clinical trials showed its efficacy and favorable safety profile on AD patients. Taking all the clinical trials together, about 70% of the patients achieved an EASI 75 or higher with a time-to-full-clinical-response of about 4 weeks. Pruritus showed a rapid response with an initial improvement at 2 weeks [71, 75].

Recent case series have observed a similar response [76].

It has been shown that dupilumab improves the AD inflammatory signature [77].

The main reported side effects were conjunctivitis and local reaction at the site of injection.

The recommended dose of dupilumab in adults is an initial dose of 600 mg followed by 300 mg every 15 days. There is no need for complementary studies before starting the treatment.

Only patients with previous helminthic infections should receive specific treatment before dupilumab.

Due to a lack of data, live and live attenuated vaccines should not be given currently with dupilumab. It is recommended to be up to date with immunization prior to the treatment. Contraindications include hypersensitivity to dupilumab or any of its excipients [78].

Currently, dupilumab is also licensed for asthma.

4.4 New treatments

Several other molecules are under investigation [70].

4.4.1 Biologicals

Tralokinumab and lebrikizumab are fully human monoclonal antibodies that target IL-13. They have shown sustained clinical improvement in moderate-to-severe AD patients in phase II studies with an acceptable safety and tolerability profile. Wollenberg et al. showed that patients with higher serum levels of periostin and DDP4 had a better response to tralokinumab compared to those with lower levels [52].

Tralokinumab has already begun phase III trials, whereas lebrikizumab has yet to start.

Nemolizumab, a humanized monoclonal antibody against the receptor A of IL-31, has also shown efficacy in phase II trials in patients with moderate-to-severe AD. IL-31 plays a role in the pathogenesis of AD and pruritus. The two phase 2 clinical trial showed not only a rapid and maintained effect on pruritus but also AD scores (EASI and BSA) [79, 80].

Fezakinumab is a fully human monoclonal antibody against IL-22. The phase 2a clinical trial showed a sustained clinical improvement in severe AD patients [81].

Tezepelumab is a fully human monoclonal antibody that targets TSLP. In the phase 2a trial, a non-statistically significant improvement over placebo at week 12 was observed [82].

There are contradictory papers regarding the efficacy of ustekinumab, a fully human monoclonal antibody against the p40 subunit shared by IL-12 and IL-23 [83–88].

4.4.2 Small molecules

There are several small molecules in development for AD.

Apremilast is an oral PDE4 inhibitor approved for the treatment of obstructive pulmonary disease, plaque psoriasis, and psoriatic arthritis [89]. Small series of cases have shown its potential as a treatment for AD [90, 91].

Baricitinib, a JAK 1 and 2 inhibitors, abrocitinib and upadacitinib, selective JAK 1 inhibitors, are currently running phase 3 trials. Phase 2 showed positive results regarding efficacy and safety for the three molecules [92].

Finally, delgocitinib, a small molecule that targets JAK 1, 2, 3 and TYK 2 demonstrated rapid improvement in clinical signs and symptoms with a favorable safety profile, in a phase 2 trial [93].

Author details

Ignasi Figueras-Nart[1*] and Oscar Palomares-Gracia[2]

1 Department of Dermatology and Venereology, Hospital Universitari de Bellvitge, L'Hospitalet de Llobregat, Barcelona, Spain

2 Department of Biochemistry and Molecular Biology, Vaccines and Dendritic Cells Lab., Chemistry School, Complutense University of Madrid, Madrid, Spain

*Address all correspondence to: ignasifiguerasnart@gmail.com

References

[1] Lifschitz C. The impact of atopic dermatitis on quality of life. Annals of Nutrition & Metabolism. 2015;**66** (Suppl 1):34-40

[2] Palomares O, Akdis M, Martín-Fontecha M, Akdis CA. Mechanisms of immune regulation in allergic diseases: The role of regulatory T and B cells. Immunological Reviews. 2017;**278**(1):219-236

[3] Palomares O, Martín-Fontecha M, Lauener R, Traidl-Hoffmann C, Cavkaytar O, Akdis M, et al. Regulatory T cells and immune regulation of allergic diseases: Roles of IL-10 and TGF-β. Genes and Immunity. 2014;**15**(8):511-520

[4] Palomares Ó, Sánchez-Ramón S, Dávila I, Prieto L, Pérez de Llano L, Lleonart M, et al. dIvergEnt: How IgE axis contributes to the continuum of allergic asthma and anti-IgE therapies. International Journal of Molecular Sciences. 2017;**18**(6)

[5] Weidinger S, Novak N. Atopic dermatitis. The Lancet. 2016;**387**(10023):1109-1122

[6] Sánchez-Ramón S, Conejero L, Netea MG, Sancho D, Palomares Ó, Subiza JL. Trained immunity-based vaccines: A new paradigm for the development of broad-spectrum anti-infectious formulations. Frontiers in Immunology. 2018;**9**:2936

[7] Czarnowicki T, Krueger JG, Guttman-Yassky E. Novel concepts of prevention and treatment of atopic dermatitis through barrier and immune manipulations with implications for the atopic march. The Journal of Allergy and Clinical Immunology. 2017;**139**(6):1723-1734

[8] Werfel T, Allam J-P, Biedermann T, Eyerich K, Gilles S, Guttman-Yassky E, et al. Cellular and molecular immunologic mechanisms in patients with atopic dermatitis. The Journal of Allergy and Clinical Immunology. 2016;**138**(2):336-349

[9] Otsuka A, Nomura T, Rerknimitr P, Seidel JA, Honda T, Kabashima K. The interplay between genetic and environmental factors in the pathogenesis of atopic dermatitis. Immunological Reviews. 2017;**278**(1):246-262

[10] Dainichi T, Kitoh A, Otsuka A, Nakajima S, Nomura T, Kaplan DH, Kabashima K. The epithelial immune microenvironment (EIME) in atopic dermatitis and psoriasis. Nature Immunology. 2018;**19**(12):1286-1298

[11] Brunner PM, Guttman-Yassky E, Leung DYM. The immunology of atopic dermatitis and its reversibility with broad-spectrum and targeted therapies. The Journal of Allergy and Clinical Immunology. 2017;**139**(4S):S65-S76

[12] Rerknimitr P, Otsuka A, Nakashima C, Kabashima K. The etiopathogenesis of atopic dermatitis: Barrier disruption, immunological derangement, and pruritus. Inflammation and Regeneration. 2017;**37**:14

[13] Gandhi NA, Bennett BL, Graham NMH, Pirozzi G, Stahl N, Yancopoulos GD. Targeting key proximal drivers of type 2 inflammation in disease. Nature Reviews. Drug Discovery. 2016;**15**(1):35-50

[14] Czarnowicki T, He H, Krueger JG, Guttman-Yassky E. Atopic dermatitis endotypes and implications for targeted therapeutics. The Journal of Allergy and Clinical Immunology. 2019;**143**(1):1-11

[15] Cabanillas B, Brehler A-C, Novak N. Atopic dermatitis phenotypes and the need for personalized medicine.

Current Opinion in Allergy and Clinical Immunology. 2017;**17**(4):309-315

[16] Galli SJ, Starkl P, Marichal T, Tsai M. Mast cells and IgE can enhance survival during innate and acquired host responses to venoms. Transactions of the American Clinical and Climatological Association. 2017;**128**:193-221

[17] Mukai K, Tsai M, Starkl P, Marichal T, Galli SJ. IgE and mast cells in host defense against parasites and venoms. Seminars in Immunopathology. 2016;**38**(5):581-603

[18] Palomares O. The role of regulatory T cells in IgE-mediated food allergy. Journal of Investigational Allergology & Clinical Immunology. 2013;**23**(6):371-382

[19] Annunziato F, Romagnani C, Romagnani S. The 3 major types of innate and adaptive cell-mediated effector immunity. The Journal of Allergy and Clinical Immunology. 2015;**135**(3):626-635

[20] Agache I, Akdis CA. Precision medicine and phenotypes, endotypes, genotypes, regiotypes, and theratypes of allergic diseases. The Journal of Clinical Investigation. 2019;**130**:1493-1503

[21] Roan F, Obata-Ninomiya K, Ziegler SF. Epithelial cell-derived cytokines: More than just signaling the alarm. The Journal of Clinical Investigation. 2019;**129**(4):1441-1451

[22] Schuijs MJ, Hammad H, Lambrecht BN. Professional and 'amateur' antigen-presenting cells in type 2 immunity. Trends in Immunology. 2019;**40**(1):22-34

[23] Novak N, Koch S, Allam J-P, Bieber T. Dendritic cells: Bridging innate and adaptive immunity in atopic dermatitis. The Journal of Allergy and Clinical Immunology. 2010;**125**(1):50-59

[24] Akdis M, Aab A, Altunbulakli C, Azkur K, Costa RA, Crameri R, et al. Interleukins (from IL-1 to IL-38), interferons, transforming growth factor β, and TNF-α: Receptors, functions, and roles in diseases. The Journal of Allergy and Clinical Immunology. 2016;**138**(4):984-1010

[25] Akdis M, Burgler S, Crameri R, Eiwegger T, Fujita H, Gomez E, et al. Interleukins, from 1 to 37, and interferon-γ: Receptors, functions, and roles in diseases. The Journal of Allergy and Clinical Immunology. 2011;**127**(3):701-721

[26] Akdis M, Palomares O, van de Veen W, van Splunter M, Akdis CA. TH17 and TH22 cells: A confusion of antimicrobial response with tissue inflammation versus protection. The Journal of Allergy and Clinical Immunology. 2012;**129**(6):1438-1449

[27] Palomares O, Yaman G, Azkur AK, Akkoc T, Akdis M, Akdis CA. Role of Treg in immune regulation of allergic diseases. European Journal of Immunology. 2010;**40**(5):1232-1240

[28] Durand M, Segura E. The known unknowns of the human dendritic cell network. Frontiers in Immunology. 2015;**6**:129

[29] Miller JC, Brown BD, Shay T, Gautier EL, Jojic V, Cohain A, et al. Deciphering the transcriptional network of the dendritic cell lineage. Nature Immunology. 2012;**13**(9):888-899

[30] Crozat K, Guiton R, Guilliams M, Henri S, Baranek T, Schwartz-Cornil I, et al. Comparative genomics as a tool to reveal functional equivalences between human and mouse dendritic cell subsets. Immunological Reviews. 2010;**234**(1):177-198

[31] Novak N. An update on the role of human dendritic cells in patients with atopic dermatitis. The Journal of Allergy and Clinical Immunology. 2012;**129**(4):879-886

[32] Feld M, Garcia R, Buddenkotte J, Katayama S, Lewis K, Muirhead G, et al. The pruritus- and TH2-associated cytokine IL-31 promotes growth of sensory nerves. The Journal of Allergy and Clinical Immunology. 2016;**138**(2):500-508

[33] Meng J, Moriyama M, Feld M, Buddenkotte J, Buhl T, Szöllösi A, et al. New mechanism underlying IL-31-induced atopic dermatitis. The Journal of Allergy and Clinical Immunology. 2018;**141**(5):1677-1689.e8

[34] Stott B, Lavender P, Lehmann S, Pennino D, Durham S, Schmidt-Weber CB. Human IL-31 is induced by IL-4 and promotes TH2-driven inflammation. The Journal of Allergy and Clinical Immunology. 2013;**132**(2):446-454.e5

[35] Sanyal RD, Pavel AB, Glickman J, Chan TC, Zheng X, Zhang N, et al. Atopic dermatitis in African American patients is TH2/TH22-skewed with TH1/TH17 attenuation. Annals of Allergy, Asthma & Immunology. 2019;**122**(1):99-110.e6

[36] Chan TC, Sanyal RD, Pavel AB, Glickman J, Zheng X, Xu H, et al. Atopic dermatitis in Chinese patients shows TH2/TH17 skewing with psoriasiform features. The Journal of Allergy and Clinical Immunology. 2018;**142**(3):1013-1017

[37] Silvestre Salvador JF, Romero-Pérez D, Encabo-Durán B. Atopic dermatitis in adults: A diagnostic challenge. Journal of Investigational Allergology & Clinical Immunology. 2017;**27**(2):78-88

[38] Bieber T. Atopic dermatitis. The New England Journal of Medicine. 2008;**358**(14):1483-1494

[39] Bieber T, D'Erme AM, Akdis CA, Traidl-Hoffmann C, Lauener R, Schäppi G, et al. Clinical phenotypes and endophenotypes of atopic dermatitis: Where are we, and where should we go? The Journal of Allergy and Clinical Immunology. 2017;**139**(4S):S58-S64

[40] Hello M, Aubert H, Bernier C, Néel A, Barbarot S. Atopic dermatitis of the adult. La Revue de Médecine Interne. 2016;**37**(2):91-99

[41] Eichenfield LF, Hanifin JM, Luger TA, Stevens SR, Pride HB. Consensus conference on pediatric atopic dermatitis. Journal of the American Academy of Dermatology. 2003;**49**(6):1088-1095

[42] Liu P, Zhao Y, Mu Z-L, Lu Q-J, Zhang L, Yao X, et al. Clinical features of adult/adolescent atopic dermatitis and Chinese criteria for atopic dermatitis. Chinese Medical Journal. 2016;**129**(7):757-762

[43] Eichenfield LF, Tom WL, Chamlin SL, Feldman SR, Hanifin JM, Simpson EL, et al. Guidelines of care for the management of atopic dermatitis: Section 1. Diagnosis and assessment of atopic dermatitis. Journal of the American Academy of Dermatology. 2014;**70**(2):338-351

[44] Hernández-Bel P, de la Cuadra J, García R, Alegre V. Protein contact dermatitis: Review of 27 cases. Actas Dermo-Sifiliográficas. 2011;**102**(5):336-343

[45] Chernyshov PV, Tomas-Aragones L, Manolache L, Marron SE, Salek MS, Poot F, et al. Quality of life measurement in atopic dermatitis. Position paper of the European academy of dermatology and venereology (EADV) task force on quality of life. Journal of the European Academy of Dermatology and Venereology. 2017;**31**(4):576-593

[46] Biomarkers In Risk Assessment: Validity And Validation (EHC 222, 2001) [Internet]. Available from: http://www.inchem.org/documents/ehc/ehc/ehc222.htm [cited August 2, 2019]

[47] Biomarkers Definitions Working Group. Biomarkers and surrogate endpoints: Preferred definitions and conceptual framework. Clinical Pharmacology and Therapeutics. 2001;**69**(3):89-95

[48] Thijs JL, de Bruin-Weller MS, Hijnen D. Current and future biomarkers in atopic dermatitis. Immunology and Allergy Clinics of North America. 2017;**37**(1):51-61

[49] Pipinić IS, Macan J. Filaggrin gene null-mutations and atopic diseases. Acta Medica Croatica. 2015;**69**(5):467-473

[50] Gao P-S, Rafaels NM, Hand T, Murray T, Boguniewicz M, Hata T, et al. Filaggrin mutations that confer risk of atopic dermatitis confer greater risk for eczema herpeticum. The Journal of Allergy and Clinical Immunology. 2009;**124**(3):507-513

[51] G A, Rasheed Z, Salama RH, Salem T, Ahmed AA, Zedan K, et al. Filaggrin, major basic protein and leukotriene B4: Biomarkers for adult patients of bronchial asthma, atopic dermatitis and allergic rhinitis. Intractable & Rare Diseases Research. 2018;**7**(4):264-270

[52] Wollenberg A, Howell MD, Guttman-Yassky E, Silverberg JI, Kell C, Ranade K, et al. Treatment of atopic dermatitis with tralokinumab, an anti-IL-13 mAb. The Journal of Allergy and Clinical Immunology. 2019;**143**(1):135-141

[53] Bloomfeld RS, Bickston SJ, Levine MM, Carroll SL . Thiopurine Methyltransferase activity is correlated with azathioprine metabolite levels in patients with inflammatory bowel disease in clinical gastroenterology practice. The Journal of Applied Research. 2006;**6**(4):282-287

[54] Thijs J, Krastev T, Weidinger S, Buckens CF, de Bruin-Weller M, Bruijnzeel-Koomen C, et al. Biomarkers for atopic dermatitis: A systematic review and meta-analysis. Current Opinion in Allergy and Clinical Immunology. 2015;**15**(5):453-460

[55] Thijs JL, Nierkens S, Herath A, CAF B-K, Knol EF, Giovannone B, et al. A panel of biomarkers for disease severity in atopic dermatitis. Clinical and Experimental Allergy. 2015;**45**(3):698-701

[56] Thijs JL, Drylewicz J, Fiechter R, Strickland I, Sleeman MA, Herath A, et al. EASI p-EASI: Utilizing a combination of serum biomarkers offers an objective measurement tool for disease severity in atopic dermatitis patients. The Journal of Allergy and Clinical Immunology. 2017;**140**(6):1703-1705

[57] Kim HS, Kim JH, Seo YM, Chun YH, Yoon J-S, Kim HH, et al. Eosinophil-derived neurotoxin as a biomarker for disease severity and relapse in recalcitrant atopic dermatitis. Annals of Allergy, Asthma & Immunology. 2017;**119**(5):441-445

[58] Kou K, Okawa T, Yamaguchi Y, Ono J, Inoue Y, Kohno M, et al. Periostin levels correlate with disease severity and chronicity in patients with atopic dermatitis. The British Journal of Dermatology. 2014;**171**(2):283-291

[59] Sahiner UM, Buyuktiryaki B, Gungor HE, Sahiner N, Turasan A, Torun YA, et al. Factors that predict disease severity in atopic dermatitis: The role of serum basal tryptase. Allergy and Asthma Proceedings. 2018;**39**(5):371-376

[60] Lee KS, Oh I-H, Choi SH, Rha Y-H. Analysis of epidemiology and risk

factors of atopic dermatitis in Korean children and adolescents from the 2010 Korean national health and nutrition examination survey. BioMed Research International. 2017;**2017**:5142754

[61] Kelleher M, Dunn-Galvin A, Hourihane JO, Murray D, Campbell LE, McLean WHI, et al. Skin barrier dysfunction measured by transepidermal water loss at 2 days and 2 months predates and predicts atopic dermatitis at 1 year. The Journal of Allergy and Clinical Immunology. 2015;**135**(4):930-935.e1

[62] O'Donovan SM, O'B Hourihane J, Murray DM, Kenny LC, Khashan AS, Chaoimh CN, et al. Neonatal adiposity increases the risk of atopic dermatitis during the first year of life. The Journal of Allergy and Clinical Immunology. 2016;**137**(1):108-117

[63] Ring J, Alomar A, Bieber T, Deleuran M, Fink-Wagner A, Gelmetti C, et al. Guidelines for treatment of atopic eczema (atopic dermatitis) part II. Journal of the European Academy of Dermatology and Venereology. 2012;**26**(9):1176-1193

[64] Shrestha S, Miao R, Wang L, Chao J, Yuce H, Wei W. Burden of atopic dermatitis in the United States: Analysis of healthcare claims data in the commercial, medicare, and medical databases. Advances in Therapy. 2017;**34**(8):1989-2006

[65] Andersen YMF, Egeberg A, Gislason GH, Hansen PR, Skov L, Thyssen JP. Risk of myocardial infarction, ischemic stroke, and cardiovascular death in patients with atopic dermatitis. The Journal of Allergy and Clinical Immunology. 2016;**138**(1):310-312

[66] Brunner PM, Suárez-Fariñas M, He H, Malik K, Wen H-C, Gonzalez J, et al. The atopic dermatitis blood signature is characterized by increases in inflammatory and cardiovascular risk proteins. Scientific Reports. 2017;7(1):8707

[67] Serra-Baldrich E, de Frutos JO, Jáuregui I, Armario-Hita JC, Silvestre JF, Herraez L, et al. Changing perspectives in atopic dermatitis. Allergol Immunopathol (Madr). 2017

[68] Wollenberg A, Barbarot S, Bieber T, Christen-Zaech S, Deleuran M, Fink-Wagner A, et al. Consensus-based European guidelines for treatment of atopic eczema (atopic dermatitis) in adults and children: Part I. Journal of the European Academy of Dermatology and Venereology. 2018;**32**(5):657-682

[69] Simpson EL, Chalmers JR, Hanifin JM, Thomas KS, Cork MJ, McLean WHI, et al. Emollient enhancement of the skin barrier from birth offers effective atopic dermatitis prevention. The Journal of Allergy and Clinical Immunology. 2014;**134**(4):818-823

[70] Deleanu D, Nedelea I. Biological therapies for atopic dermatitis: An update. Experimental and Therapeutic Medicine. 2019;**17**(2):1061-1067

[71] Wollenberg A, Barbarot S, Bieber T, Christen-Zaech S, Deleuran M, Fink-Wagner A, et al. Consensus-based European guidelines for treatment of atopic eczema (atopic dermatitis) in adults and children: Part II. Journal of the European Academy of Dermatology and Venereology. 2018;**32**(6):850-878

[72] Eckert L, Amand C, Gadkari A, Rout R, Hudson R, Ardern-Jones M. Treatment patterns in UK adult patients with atopic dermatitis treated with systemic immunosuppressants: Data from the health improvement network (THIN). Journal of Dermatological Treatment. 2019;**15**:1-6

[73] Roekevisch E, Schram ME, Leeflang MMG, Brouwer MWD,

Gerbens LAA, Bos JD, et al. Methotrexate versus azathioprine in patients with atopic dermatitis: 2-year follow-up data. The Journal of Allergy and Clinical Immunology. 2018;**141**(2):825-827

[74] Schram ME, Roekevisch E, Leeflang MMG, Bos JD, Schmitt J, Spuls PI. A randomized trial of methotrexate versus azathioprine for severe atopic eczema. The Journal of Allergy and Clinical Immunology. 2011;**128**(2):353-359

[75] Simpson EL, Bieber T, Guttman-Yassky E, Beck LA, Blauvelt A, Cork MJ, et al. Two phase 3 trials of dupilumab versus placebo in atopic dermatitis. The New England Journal of Medicine. 2016;**375**(24):2335-2348

[76] Armario-Hita JC, Pereyra-Rodriguez J, Silvestre JF, Ruiz-VillaverdeR, ValeroA, Izu-BellosoR, et al. Treatment of moderate-to-severe atopic dermatitis with dupilumab in real clinical practice: A multicentre, retrospective case series. The British Journal of Dermatology. 2019:25

[77] Hamilton JD, Suárez-Fariñas M, Dhingra N, Cardinale I, Li X, Kostic A, et al. Dupilumab improves the molecular signature in skin of patients with moderate-to-severe atopic dermatitis. The Journal of Allergy and Clinical Immunology. 2014;**134**(6):1293-1300

[78] DUPIXENT (dupilumab) injection. European Medicines Agency; 2017

[79] Ruzicka T, Lynde CW, Jemec GBE, Diepgen T, Berth-Jones J, Coenraads PJ, et al. Efficacy and safety of oral alitretinoin (9-cis retinoic acid) in patients with severe chronic hand eczema refractory to topical corticosteroids: Results of a randomized, double-blind, placebo-controlled, multicentre trial. The British Journal of Dermatology. 2008;**158**(4):808-817

[80] Kabashima K, Furue M, Hanifin JM, Pulka G, Wollenberg A, Galus R, et al. Nemolizumab in patients with moderate-to-severe atopic dermatitis: Randomized, phase II, long-term extension study. The Journal of Allergy and Clinical Immunology. 2018;**142**(4):1121-1130

[81] Guttman-Yassky E, Brunner PM, Neumann AU, Khattri S, Pavel AB, Malik K, et al. Efficacy and safety of fezakinumab (an IL-22 monoclonal antibody) in adults with moderate-to-severe atopic dermatitis inadequately controlled by conventional treatments: A randomized, double-blind, phase 2a trial. Journal of the American Academy of Dermatology. 2018;**78**(5):872-881

[82] Simpson EL, Parnes JR, She D, Crouch S, Rees W, Mo M, et al. Tezepelumab, an anti-thymic stromal lymphopoietin monoclonal antibody, in the treatment of moderate to severe atopic dermatitis: A randomized phase 2a clinical trial. Journal of the American Academy of Dermatology. 2019;**80**(4):1013-1021

[83] Samuel RJ, Reynolds NJ. Ustekinumab for severe atopic dermatitis: An important negative study. The British Journal of Dermatology. 2017;**177**(2):339-341

[84] Pan Y, Xu L, Qiao J, Fang H. A systematic review of ustekinumab in the treatment of atopic dermatitis. Journal of Dermatological Treatment. 2018;**29**(6):539-541

[85] Ishiuji Y, Umezawa Y, Asahina A, Fukuta H, Aizawa N, Yanaba K, et al. Exacerbation of atopic dermatitis symptoms by ustekinumab in psoriatic patients with elevated serum immunoglobulin E levels: Report of

two cases. The Journal of Dermatology. 2018;**45**(6):732-734

[86] Agusti-Mejias A, Messeguer F, García R, Febrer I. Severe refractory atopic dermatitis in an adolescent patient successfully treated with ustekinumab. Annals of Dermatology. 2013;**25**(3):368-370

[87] Shroff A, Guttman-Yassky E. Successful use of ustekinumab therapy in refractory severe atopic dermatitis. JAAD Case Reports. 2015;**1**(1):25-26

[88] Puya R, Alvarez-López M, Velez A, Casas Asuncion E, Moreno JC. Treatment of severe refractory adult atopic dermatitis with ustekinumab. International Journal of Dermatology. 2012;**51**(1):115-116

[89] Dastidar SG, Rajagopal D, Ray A. Therapeutic benefit of PDE4 inhibitors in inflammatory diseases. Current Opinion in Investigational Drugs. 2007;**8**(5):364-372

[90] Abrouk M, Farahnik B, Zhu TH, Nakamura M, Singh R, Lee K, et al. Apremilast treatment of atopic dermatitis and other chronic eczematous dermatoses. Journal of the American Academy of Dermatology. 2017;**77**(1):177-180

[91] Samrao A, Berry TM, Goreshi R, Simpson EL. A pilot study of an oral phosphodiesterase inhibitor (apremilast) for atopic dermatitis in adults. Archives of Dermatology. 2012;**148**(8):890-897

[92] Cotter DG, Schairer D, Eichenfield L. Emerging therapies for atopic dermatitis: JAK inhibitors. Journal of the American Academy of Dermatology. 2018;**78**(3, Suppl 1):S53-S62

[93] Nakagawa H, Nemoto O, Igarashi A, Nagata T. Efficacy and safety of topical JTE-052, a Janus kinase inhibitor, in Japanese adult patients with moderate-to-severe atopic dermatitis: A phase II, multicentre, randomized, vehicle-controlled clinical study. The British Journal of Dermatology. 2018;**178**(2):424-432

Chapter 3

Epigenetic Studies of Atopic Dermatitis

Vladimir Sobolev, Elizaveta Bystritskaya and Oxana Svitich

Abstract

Since the pathogenesis of atopic dermatitis could not be explained only by a population genetic and phenotypic profiles, epigenetic regulator factors have been considered. Epigenetics is the study of inherited changes in gene expression that are not related to changes in its nucleotide sequence. One of the main classical regulatory mechanisms in human cells is DNA methylation. It is not clear how permanent modifications caused by this process are and whether it is possible to affect them by changing the activity of enzymes that trigger remodeling reactions. In this chapter we analyze all recent studies in this field. We focus more on methylation of innate and adaptive immune factors, with an emphasis on T-lymphocyte genes such as CD3, CD4, and CD8.

Keywords: atopic dermatitis, epigenetics, DNA methylation, genome-wide methylation analysis, immune system

1. Introduction

Atopic dermatitis (AD) is a chronic recurrent inflammation of the skin, characterized by impairment of the epidermal barrier that entailing its further dysfunction. The predisposition to IgE-mediated hypertension contributes to such a malfunction, realized in sensitization to surrounding allergens [1]. This pathology is also characterized by infiltration and accumulation of type 2 T helper cells (Th2) and eosinophils [2]. Atopic dermatitis is a multifactorial disease. The main triggers are various genetically predetermined defects of the epidermal barrier and the immune system influenced by environment [1].

Thus, the study of tissues and cells transcriptome involved in the pathogenesis of the disease is one of the best options for detecting molecular signs of complex diseases such as AD [3]. In one of these studies, it was found that the expression of a large number of genes which were responsible for terminal differentiation of keratinocytes was reduced in case of AD compared with healthy controls. These genes include filaggrin (*FLG*), loricrin (*LOR*), involucrin, late cornified envelope protein *LCE2B*, and genes encoding the S100 family of proteins [4]. This study showed that AD is associated with impaired keratinization processes in the epidermis, and confirmed another profile study by Sugiura et al., where suppression of *LOR* and *FLG* expression was determined in the lesional skin [5]. With the help of RNA sequencing technology by which transcriptomes of intact and damaged skin of patients with moderate and severe AD were compared, an increased expression of

 IntechOpen

the *TREM-1* signaling pathway, as well as *IL-36*, was revealed [6]. The laser capture microdissection method once again confirmed that the expression of genes encoding skin barrier proteins, including *FLG*, *LOR*, *CLDN4* and *CLDN8*, is reduced in affected atopic skin; and, on the contrary, the expression of cytokines Th2 and Th17 genes, such as *CCL22*, *CCL26*, *TSLP*, and *IL-22* etc., is increased [7].

Loss of function mutations in the gene encoding *FLG* are one of the most significant genetic risk factors for AD. A transcriptome profiling study realized by RNA sequencing revealed differentially expressed genes involved in the extracellular reactions, lipid metabolism, and stress response. In FLG-deficient skin, the stress response mediated by type I interferon (IFN) was expressed [8].

However, genetic changes solely do not fully shed light on the molecular mechanisms involved in the pathogenesis of AD. Therefore, epigenetic mechanisms involved in the genomic adaptation according to environmental conditions may possibly explain how environmental exposure affects the risk of allergy development.

Epigenetic mechanisms, in particular methylation, play a key role in immune regulation and are influenced by a variety of environmental factors leading to persistent molecular changes in genes. The methylation process involves the addition of a methyl group to the cytosine (C5 position; 5-methylcytosine, 5mC). DNA methylation occurs primarily in the context of CpG dinucleotides and is the main epigenetic modification involved in the regulation of chromatin structure and gene expression [9].

2. Targeted methylation studies

2.1 DNA methyltransferase studies

The main enzymes responsible for the methylation process in humans are DNA methyltransferases 1, 3a, and 3b (DNMT1, DNMT3a, and DNMT3b). It is generally accepted that DNMT3a and DNMT3b are *de novo* methyltransferases that form a model of DNA methylation at early stages of development, as well as its changes during cell differentiation [10]. DNA methyltransferase 1 (DNMT1) maintains the methylated state of DNA by attaching methyl groups to one of the DNA strands at the sites where the other complementary strand is methylated [9].

In the context of the AD study, only DNA methyltransferase-1 (DNMT-1), an enzyme that catalyzes the methylation of cytosine bases in CpG islands, has so far been considered. Nakamura et al. for the first time carried out an indirect assessment of methylation status in patients with atopic dermatitis by measuring the expression of messenger RNA (mRNA) of DNA methyltransferase-1 in peripheral blood mononuclear cells (PBMC) by quantitative RT-PCR. Although the expression level of *DNMT-1* mRNA had a tendency to decrease in patients with atopic dermatitis compared with healthy controls, there were no significant differences between these groups [11]. However, in the group of patients with AD, the IgE level was also taken into account. It was found that the level of *DNMT-1* mRNA was significantly lower in the high IgE group compared to the control group.

It is common knowledge that many local factors, such as skin impairment, play an important role in the development of AD [12, 13]. However, Th2-infiltration in response to penetration of allergens and production of cytokines by infiltrated cells (for example, IL-4 and IL-5) plays the key role in the development of IgE-mediated response and chronic inflammation involving eosinophils [14–16]. It is assumed that in these processes DNA hypomethylation contributes to the hyperreactivity of Th2 cells in response to allergens and, as a consequence, cytokine-mediated

IgE production. It has also been suggested that IL-4-mediated IgE production in patients with high serum IgE levels is associated with DNA hypomethylation in B cells [16, 17]. In this study the decrease in *DNMT-1* expression in PBMCs in patients with high IgE levels also confirmed the concept that AD is promoted by lower *DNMT-1* levels.

On the other hand, the lack of significant differences while comparing *DNMT-1* expression between groups with high and low IgE levels, along with no correlation between *DNMT-1* expression and serum IgE levels in the respective patients, indicates that *DNMT-1* cannot be a factor that solely affects serum IgE. To clarify this issue, more studies are needed in which *DMNT-1* levels would be assessed in patients without AD but with high serum IgE levels.

2.2 *FCER1G* methylation studies

Based on the opinion that overexpression of the high-affinity IgE receptor on monocytes and dendritic cells contributes to the pathogenesis of AD, a group of scientists studied the epigenetic mechanism of deregulation of high-affinity IgE receptors – FcεRI [18].

Liang et al. measured the methylation level of total DNA of monocytes from 10 patients with AD and 10 healthy people from the control group. Bisulfite sequencing was used as the main method to determine the methylation status of the *FCER1G* promoter region. To determine the functional significance of methylation changes in FcεRI expression, targeted methylation of the sequence and a demethylating agent, 5-azacytidine (5-aza), were used. The levels of FcεRIγ mRNA and FcεRI protein were determined using RT-PCR RT, Western blotting, and flow cytometry, respectively.

Thus, total hypomethylation in $CD14^+$ monocytes in patients with AD was revealed, as well as locus-specific hypomethylation of the *FCER1G* promoter region in comparison with healthy controls. In addition, hypomethylation of *FCER1G* contributed to its increased expression. Targeted methylation in combination with a reporter luciferase assay confirmed this association between methylation and expression. Moreover, treatment of monocytes of healthy people with 5-azacytidine caused a decrease in methylation levels and induction of FcεRIγ transcription and expression of surface FcεRI. The authors showed that demethylation of specific regulatory elements at the *FCER1G* locus promotes an increase in FcεRI expression in monocytes in patients with AD, which, in turn, leads to an enhanced allergic response.

Atopic monocytes with high FcεRI levels are thought to play an important role in the pathogenesis of AD. This is due to the fact that monocytes carrying FcεRI can differentiate into inflammatory dendritic epidermal cells (IDECs), which intensify allergic inflammatory reactions in the skin by stimulating T cells, and are also involved in the transition to the chronic course of AD with a predominance of Th2 [19, 20]. In this study, it was shown for the first time that changes in the epigenetic regulation of the *FCER1G* gene can explain the pathological activation of FcεRI on patient monocytes.

2.3 *TSLP methylation studies*

Thymic stromal lymphopoietin (TSLP) plays an important role in maintaining T-cell homeostasis and, apparently, is of great importance in the development of allergic symptoms, especially in atopic dermatitis and asthma [21, 22]. Human TSLP is overexpressed in keratinocytes of patients with acute and chronic AD. However, the mechanism of such TSLP expression remains unclear. The question is whether

TSLP expression is regulated by modification of aberrant DNA methylation of *TSLP* promoter in keratinocytes of AD patients [23].

It is known that the TSLP protein cannot be found in healthy skin, in skin lesions in patients with nickel contact dermatitis or in patients with disseminated lupus erythematosus, as well as in intact skin in patients with AD; however, increased levels of TSLP expression are observed in both acute and chronic atopic skin lesions [21, 24]. TSLP overexpression in keratinocytes can activate myeloid dendritic cells by enhancing the surface expression of CD54, CD80, CD83, CD86 molecules and MHC class II molecules on myeloid dendritic cells [25], which lead to Th2-inflammatory reactions [24].

Luo et al. measured the levels of mRNA and TSLP protein in samples of affected skin from 10 atopic children and 10 healthy people from the control group, using quantitative RT-PCR and immunohistochemistry [26]. Bisulfite sequencing was performed to determine the methylation status of the *TSLP* promoter; 5-aza, a DNA methyltransferase inhibitor, was used to determine the effect of DNA methylation on TSLP expression.

As a result, the levels of expression of mRNA and TSLP protein relative to β-actin were significantly higher in affected skin regions of patients with AD compared with healthy controls. In addition, hypomethylation of the promoter region of the *TSLP* gene containing 16 CG pairs was found in the affected skin regions. Upon treatment of HaCaT cell line keratinocytes with 5-aza, the methylation level of the *TSLP* promoter decreased significantly, while its transcription increased.

It can be concluded that DNA demethylation of the specific regulatory region of the *TSLP* gene may contribute to the overexpression of TSLP in the affected skin regions in atopic patients. This suggests that aberrant epigenetic modifications play an important role in the pathogenesis of this disease.

In another study, the authors tried to reveal the effect of prenatal smoking on DNA methylation in case of atopic disorders [27]. Methylation differences associated with exposure to tobacco smoke were initially identified with the use of Illumina Infinium 27 K methylation kits in 14 children in a Taiwanese study cohort. Information on the course of the disease and possible risk factors was collected. Cord blood levels of cotinine were measured in order to represent prenatal smoking. CpG loci, in which statistically significant differences in methylation were found, were validated by methylation-dependent fragment separation (MDFS). Differential methylation in three genes (*TSLP*, *GSTT1*, and *CYB5R3*) was detected during the experiment. Among these, only the *TSLP* gene showed a significant difference in the percentage of promoter methylation after testing with MDFS. The *TSLP* gene was further investigated in a larger sample group (150 children) which completed a follow-up study. The *TSLP* 5'-CpG island (5'CGI) methylation status has been found to be significantly associated with prenatal exposure to smoke and atopic dermatitis. The degree of the *TSLP* 5'CGI methylation was inversely correlated with the expression levels of the TSLP protein.

Thus, it can be assumed that changes in *TSLP* 5'CGI methylation decrease the regulatory function of the immune system and cause the development of Th2-type allergic inflammation in case of atopic dermatitis. The methylation status of *TSLP* 5'CGI was also found to differ depending on cotinine levels, and hypomethylated *TSLP* 5'CGI was positively associated with atopic dermatitis. Moreover, the degree of *TSLP* 5'CGI methylation and the level of TSLP protein showed an inverse correlation. This means that severe exposure to smoke can lead to *TSLP* 5'CGI hypomethylation. Therefore, hypomethylated *TSLP* 5'CGI is associated with increased gene expression and increased TSLP protein concentration. An increased level of TSLP protein may also activate Langerhans epidermal cells, contributing to the AD development. *TSLP* was also highly expressed in the lesional skin of atopic patients [24].

The results of Wang et al. study suggest that prenatal exposure to tobacco smoke is associated with a risk of atopic dermatitis, possibly through DNA methylation.

2.4 *MICAL3* methylation studies

Cho et al. conducted a research to assess the role of 25-hydroxyvitamin D (25[OH]D) deficiency in cord blood in comparison with postnatal 25[OH]D levels in AD development during the first 3 years of life and found out how 25[OH]D deficiency affects the DNA methylation profile of cord blood leukocytes [28].

Severe 25[OH]D deficiency in cord blood was associated with a higher risk of atopic dermatitis diagnosing precisely at the age from 2 to 3. Comparison of differentially methylated CpG sites in accordance with moderate and insufficient 25[OH]D levels in cord blood revealed the common *MICAL3* gene for groups with and without pathology. *MICAL3* was hypomethylated in the case of low 25[OH]D levels.

Since *MICAL3* is a member of the MICAL family of flavoprotein monooxygenases involved in axon control and actin remodeling through oxidation of its molecules or production of reactive oxygen species (ROS) [29], ROS, induced by increased expression of *MICAL3*, can then suppress the antioxidant defense of the fetus, leading to subsequent AD development during the first 3 years of life. This process probably also affects the severity of the disease, since a correlation has been established between the expression of *MICAL3* mRNA and the severity index of atopic dermatitis. In addition, *MICAL3* expression levels were associated with 25[OH]D levels in cord blood regardless of the presence of AD.

To reproduce the mechanism of atopic dermatitis associated with ROS, using the example of *MICAL3*, another gene was chosen, 8-oxoguanine-DNA glycosylase (*OGG1*), which, as is known from data on mRNA expression, contributes to the development of allergic diseases in combination with oxidative stress reactions [30]. Accordingly, in atopic children with 25[OH]D deficiency in cord blood, the expression of *OGG1* mRNA was 5.22 times higher than in healthy children with a sufficient level of 25[OH]D. *OGG1* expression levels were found to be inversely related to 25[OH]D levels and atopic dermatitis severity index. In addition, there is a significant correlation between the expression levels of *MICAL3* and *OGG1*. However, studies showing that *MICAL3* and *OGG1* are directly related have not yet been conducted.

2.5 *HBD-1* methylation studies

Noh et al. described patterns of DNA methylation of human β-defensin-1 (HBD-1), a unique antimicrobial peptide expressed in various tissues, including the skin [31]. HBD-1 may be associated with a variety of innate immune system defects in the AD pathogenesis. A possible mechanism for the decrease in *HBD-1* gene expression in atopic dermatitis was investigated, and the *HBD-1* transcription restoration in undifferentiated normal epidermal keratinocytes after treatment with a DNA methyltransferase inhibitor was shown.

Suppression of *HBD-1* in undifferentiated NHEK cells has been shown to be regulated by an epigenetic inactivation mechanism involving methylation of DNA 14 CpG dinucleotide in the 5′-region of *HBD-1*. In dermatitis-affected skin, the frequency of methylation at the CpG 3 and CpG 4 sites within the *HBD-1* promoter was significantly higher than in healthy skin.

To identify specific CpG sites that play a significant role in HBD-1 expression in NHEK cells, bisulfite genomic sequencing of the region upstream of the proximal site of the *HBD-1* promoter was performed and methylation profiles of 6 CpG dinucleotides (from CpG 3 to CpG 8) were determined. Since the single nucleotide polymorphism (rs2978863) is located at the CpG 8 locus within the *HBD-1* promoter region (GenBank accession no. NC_000008.11) in the NHEK cell line, the other five CpG dinucleotides (CpG 3–7) were subjected to bisulfite sequencing analysis. Studying the methylation profile of the *HBD-1* promoter revealed detectable demethylation at the CpG 3 and CpG 4 loci in 2-deoxy-5-azacytidine-treated NHEK cells compared with untreated control cells. Such differentially methylated single CpG units in the *HBD-1* promoter may play a special role in the regulation of *HBD-1* transcription of the NHEK cell line.

Thus, epigenetic modulation of the *HBD-1* promoter, that is, DNA methylation in two separate CpG units, can affect *HBD-1* expression *in vitro*. In the affected skin, both CpG sites were hypermethylated. The failure of skin innate immunity leading to increased colonization of *S. aureus* in atopic patients may be due to an epigenetic predisposition of constitutively expressed *HBD-1*.

3. Genome-wide DNA methylation

3.1 In naive $CD4^+$

Both atopic dermatitis and psoriasis are characterized by a targeted immune response via polarized $CD4^+$ T cells. During the polarization of naive $CD4^+$ T cells, DNA methylation plays an important role in the regulation of gene transcription. Taken into consideration the similarity of immune response of atopic dermatitis and psoriasis, Han et al. conducted a study of the global DNA methylation profile in naive $CD4^+$ T cells in patients with AD and psoriasis, as well as in healthy people using the ChIP-seq method. DNA hypomethylation (more than 4 times) was found in T-cell samples isolated from patients with psoriasis and healthy people in 26 genome sites ranging in size from 10 to 70 kb. These regions were mostly pericentromeric on 10 different chromosomes and randomly overlaid with various defining epigenome signals, such as histone modifications and binding sites for transcription factors (according to the ENCODE project), which implied the potential influence of epigenetic regulation in the development of psoriasis [32].

To determine whether naive $CD4^+$ T cells from patients with AD or psoriasis have DNA methylation patterns different from those of healthy people, complex genome-wide CpG methylation profiling was performed. The uniquely mapped regions coincided with strong histone modification signals such as H3K4Me1, H3K27Ac, and H3K4Me3, as well as with transcription factor binding sites in various cell lines.

It appears that hypomethylation in some pericentromeric regions of naive $CD4^+$ T cells may be a sign of psoriasis, but not atopic dermatitis. It is not yet clear what exact role epigenetic changes of these regions play in the development of T cells. However, these data show for the first time the importance of such changes in the development of immune-mediated skin diseases [33].

The X chromosome encodes many of immune genes, which show a higher hypermethylation pattern than other genes. It is known that abnormalities, such as inactivation of the X chromosome, can contribute to the impairment of self-structures recognition and, ultimately, lead to autoimmunity [34]. In addition, DNA methylation is involved in the initiation of the X chromosome inactivation, as well as in the stable maintenance of the gene silencing state [35]. These studies suggest that DNA methylation may affect gene expression on the X chromosome or the development of T cells in psoriasis. It was found that DNA methylation is dramatically increased in the promoter region of genes on the X chromosome in patients with psoriasis. The binding sites for CDPCR3, GATA3, BRN2, and other transcription factors were identified as slightly enriched. The data obtained on epigenome changes in T cells show that naive CD4$^+$ T cells may be involved in the development of atopic dermatitis or psoriasis even before antigenic stimulation. This may be due to the effects of various environmental factors.

3.2 Tissue-specific patterns

To determine the tissue-specific differences in DNA methylation associated with AD, the research group of Rodriguez et al. examined the DNA of whole blood, T cells, B cells, as well as the affected and unaffected epidermis of atopic patients and healthy people from the control group [36]. To identify functional associations, they studied the expression profiles of epidermal mRNA.

Whole-genome methylation analysis was performed using Human Methylation27 BeadCheap. The results for epidermal tissue were different from those for blood cells. To determine the intraindividual and interindividual differences in DNA methylation, the researchers identified a pairwise correlation of methylated regions in the same tissue in samples from patients of similar sex and age, as well as between different tissues in the same person. In whole blood, T cells, and B cells, there were no significant differences in genome DNA methylation in the pathology group as compared with and the control group, and in general, intraindividual differences in DNA methylation were greater than those between individuals. A clear link was shown in case of comparing similar tissue in different individuals for different CpG sites, which partially correlated with altered levels of gene transcripts, mainly related to the processes of epidermal differentiation (*S100A* genes) and reactions of the innate immune response - thus, this study confirms the high the level of tissue specificity for DNA methylation patterns.

Regarding differentially methylated CpG islands in the epidermal tissue, 9 regions were identified as reliably associated with atopic dermatitis: in the *CFLAR*, *GPR55*, *MMP7*, *LOC283487*, *SH2D2A*, and *ERP27* genes, these regions were hypo-methylated, and in the *LRRC8C*, *S100A5*, and *EBP49* genes, these regions were hypermethylated.

Based on analysis of whole genome mRNA expression (using HumanHT-12v3 Expression BeadChip), significant differences were revealed in seven transcripts when comparing samples of the affected skin of patients with AD and the skin of healthy people.

From nine selected pairs of differentially methylated regions / differentially expressed transcripts using the EpiTYPER system and quantitative PCR, the following combinations associated with the development of AD were successfully validated: *KRT6A/KRT6A* and *KRT6A/KRT6B* (encode keratin); *IFI27/IFI27*, *OAS2/OAS2* (belong to the family of proteins regulated by IFN), *GDPD3/GDPD3* and *S100A5/S100A2*. In most of these pairs, an inverse correlation was observed, that is, higher levels of methylation were associated with lower expression of the relevant gene, and vice versa. Such dependence is usually observed in CpG islands near the sites of transcription initiation, where DNA methylation is associated with prolonged silencing of the relevant gene.

Olisova et al. carried out a genome-wide study of DNA methylation using the Illumina Infinium Human Methylation450 BeadChip technology [37]. When comparing the affected and unaffected skin areas in atopic patients, no difference in the methylation profile was found. This suggests that epigenetic changes affected the entire skin as a whole, although they have not yet appeared in clinically intact skin areas. However, when comparing the affected skin with the skin of healthy volunteers, differentially methylated genes of the TSS200 and TSS1500 regions were isolated, whose protein products were involved in the pathogenesis of atopic dermatitis and related processes: steroid hormone biosynthesis and cell metabolism (*HSD17B14*, *HSD17B*), epithelial differentiation (*KRT31*, *LCE3D*), regulation of DNA-dependent transcription and RNA processing (*DMBX1*, *MTO1*, *SNORD93*, *WDR36*), immune response and activation of lymphocytes (*AIM2*, *CD300E*, *CLEC1A*, *DEFB135*, *IL23A*), activation of transforming growth factor β1 (*LTBP1*), cellular proliferation and apoptosis (*SERPINB3*, *EPR1*).

3.3 Replicated methylation

Another genome-wide epigenetic study examined differences in DNA methylation in atopic dermatitis together with herpetic eczema (HE), and revealed how methylation changes in patients with atopic dermatitis, complicated or uncomplicated HE [38].

490 significantly differentially methylated CpG sites were identified. Many of these were associated with indicators of disease severity, especially with the level of eosinophils (431/490 sites). One CpG region was replicated and was significantly differentially methylated based severity and phenotype.

The authors found replication for one CpG region associated with total serum IgE in the *IL4* gene, as well as possible replication for four CpG regions associated with HE in the *IL13* and *IL4* genes. It has also been shown that eosinophil levels play an important role in methylation patterns in people with AD, which via molecular mechanisms can lead to phenotypic changes.

4. Epigenetic regulation of immune system factors

It is known that abnormal epigenetic regulation of immune factors and skin barriers contribute to the pathogenesis of AD. During the development of immune system cells, epigenetic mechanisms are involved in specific changes in the variants of immune response [39]. Here are some examples.

Regulatory T cells (Tregs) play an important role in early immune programming and the formation of an adequate immune response in relation to pro-allergic or tolerant conditions. Tregs are best characterized by the expression of transcription factor 3 (Foxp3), which is important for the induction and stability of Tregs [40]. Foxp3 is controlled by DNA methylation of its transcriptional regulatory regions. Naturally induced by TGF-β Foxp3$^+$ Tregs indicate stable expression of Foxp3, which is associated with selective demethylation of an evolutionarily conserved element at the Foxp3 locus - a Treg-specific demethylated region. Inhibition of DNA methylation by azacytidine, even in the absence of exogenous TGF-β, not only promotes induction of Foxp3 expression *de novo* during priming, but also ensures stability of Foxp3 expression upon restimulation. Importantly, stable Foxp3 expression was detected only in cells with an increased level of TSDR demethylation [41]. Research suggests that prenatal environmental factors can alter DNA methylation at the *FOXP3* locus in cord blood. Babies with low Tregs identified by TSDR demethylation at birth may have a higher risk of AD developing or sensitization to food allergens in the first 3 years of life [42].

In the neonatal immune system, epigenetic regulation can be shifted away from Th1-mediated immunity in order to prevent dangerous cellular immune responses to the developing fetus. The IFN-γ gene (*IFNG*), a prototype Th1 cytokine gene whose activity is regulated during fetal development, is hypermethylated in the promoter regions of resting neonatal CD4$^+$ cells compared to adult ones [43]. Similarly, the availability of chromatin at the *TBX21* locus, a major regulator of Th1 clone committing, is attenuated in neonatal CD4$^+$ cells compared to mature cells, and a decrease of transcription factor level in peripheral T cells suppresses IFN-γ production [44]. After birth, exposure to a variety of microorganisms and the formation of microbiota contributes to the essential activation of Th1 immune responses through epigenetic modifications. In a mouse model it was shown that prenatal administration of gram-negative bacteria leads to histone H4 acetylation at the *IFNG* gene and the associated increase in IFN-γ production in the offspring [45].

MicroRNAs (miRNAs) are short, single-stranded RNA molecules that function with their associated proteins and cause the degradation of targeted mRNAs, inhibiting their translation. miRNAs play an important role in a wide range of biological processes, including proliferation, differentiation, determination of cell development, apoptosis, signal transduction, and organ development. Some miRNAs are expressed specifically for each type of cells and tissues and contribute to the maintenance of cell identity. Tissue-specific miRNAs function at various levels of gene regulation, ranging from control of targeted effector genes, incompatible with the differentiated state, to control over the levels of transcriptional regulators and alternative pre-mRNA splicing. This multilevel regulation of miRNAs influences the gene expression program of differentiated cells [46]. miRNAs, including miR-21, miR-146, and miR-223, activated in patients with allergic disorders, are also activated in the skin of patients with AD [47]. A study by Herberth et al. showed that maternal exposure to tobacco during pregnancy correlated with high levels of miRNA-223 and low Treg cell levels, which predisposed children to atopic dermatitis during the first 3 years of life [48]. Sonkoly et al. found that miR-155 was one of the most activated miRNAs in lesional skin samples from atopic patients in comparison with skin samples from healthy people. It has been found that local exposure of relevant allergens to intact skin of patients with AD induces miR-155 expression. miR-155 suppresses cytotoxic T lymphocyte – associated protein 4 - CTLA-4, which negatively regulates the function of T cells. This suppression of CTLA-4, in turn, enhances the T cell proliferative response, which can then lead to a long-term chronic inflammatory state [47].

5. Conclusion

There is not much evidence on the role of epigenetic mechanisms of innate and adaptive immunity regulation in the pathogenesis of atopic diseases, as these mechanisms have been studied recently. The described candidate genes involved in pathological processes such as dysfunction of the epidermal barrier, enhanced transmission of Th2 immunity signals, weakened innate immune responses, etc. play an important role in the pathogenesis of AD. Epigenetic studies also indicate modifications in genes involved in these mechanisms. Dysfunction of the epithelial barrier and immune response reactions together trigger the development of atopic dermatitis.

New insights on epigenetic and immunological markers associated with the risk of development of atopic dermatitis will help to create new prognostic approaches in the management of patients with atopic pathology. In this regard, it is important to have a complete understanding of the pathogenic mechanisms of an allergic disease.

Conflict of interest

The authors declare no conflict of interest.

Author details

Vladimir Sobolev[1,2*], Elizaveta Bystritskaya[1] and Oxana Svitich[1,3]

1 I. Mechnikov Research Institute for Vaccines and Sera, Moscow, Russian Federation

2 Center for Theoretical Problems of Physico-Chemical Pharmacology, RAS Moscow, Russian Federation

3 Sechenov University, Moscow, Russian Federation

*Address all correspondence to: vlsobolew@gmail.com

References

[1] Martin MJ, Estravís M, García-Sánchez A, et al. Genetics and Epigenetics of Atopic Dermatitis: An Updated Systematic Review. *Genes* 2020 ; 11: 442.

[2] Sacchetti B, Funari A, Michienzi S, et al. Self-Renewing Osteoprogenitors in Bone Marrow Sinusoids Can Organize a Hematopoietic Microenvironment. *Cell* 2007; 131: 324-336.

[3] Bin L, Leung DYM. Genetic and epigenetic studies of atopic dermatitis. *Allergy Asthma Clin Immunol* 2016; 12: 52.

[4] Guttman-Yassky E, Suárez-Fariñas M, Chiricozzi A, et al. Broad defects in epidermal cornification in atopic dermatitis identified through genomic analysis. *Journal of Allergy and Clinical Immunology* 2009; 124: 1235-1244.e58.

[5] Sugiura H, Ebise H, Tazawa T, et al. Large-scale DNA microarray analysis of atopic skin lesions shows overexpression of an epidermal differentiation gene cluster in the alternative pathway and lack of protective gene expression in the cornified envelope. *British Journal of Dermatology* 2005; 152: 146-149.

[6] Suárez-Fariñas M, Ungar B, Correa da Rosa J, et al. RNA sequencing atopic dermatitis transcriptome profiling provides insights into novel disease mechanisms with potential therapeutic implications. *Journal of Allergy and Clinical Immunology* 2015; 135: 1218-1227.

[7] Esaki H, Ewald DA, Ungar B, et al. Identification of novel immune and barrier genes in atopic dermatitis by means of laser capture microdissection. *Journal of Allergy and Clinical Immunology* 2015; 135: 153-163.

[8] Cole C, Kroboth K, Schurch NJ, et al. Filaggrin-stratified transcriptomic analysis of pediatric skin identifies mechanistic pathways in patients with atopic dermatitis. *Journal of Allergy and Clinical Immunology* 2014; 134: 82-91.

[9] Hamidi T, Singh AK, Chen T. Genetic alterations of DNA methylation machinery in human diseases. *Epigenomics* 2015; 7: 247-265.

[10] Zhang J, Yang C, Wu C, et al. DNA Methyltransferases in Cancer: Biology, Paradox, Aberrations, and Targeted Therapy. *Cancers* 2020; 12: 2123.

[11] Nakamura T, Sekigawa I, Ogasawara H, et al. Expression of DNMT-1 in patients with atopic dermatitis. *Arch Dermatol Res* 2006; 298: 253-256.

[12] Ogawa H, Yoshiike T. A speculative view of atopic dermatitis: barrier dysfunction in pathogenesis. *Journal of Dermatological Science* 1993; 5: 197-204.

[13] Sekigawa I, Yoshiike T, Iida N, et al. Allergic diseases in systemic lupus erythematosus: prevalence and immunological considerations. *Clin Exp Rheumatol* 2003; 21: 117-121.

[14] Hamid Q, Boguniewicz M, Leung DY. Differential in situ cytokine gene expression in acute versus chronic atopic dermatitis. *J Clin Invest* 1994; 94: 870-876.

[15] Reijsen FC, Wijburg OLC, Gebhardt M, et al. Different growth factor requirements for human Th2 cells may reflect in vivo induced anergy. *Clinical & Experimental Immunology* 2008; 98: 151-157.

[16] Kuwabara N, Kondo N, Fukutomi O, et al. METHYLATION PATTERNS OF I ? REGION IN B CELLS STIMULATED WITH INTERLEUKIN 4 AND EPSTEIN-BARR VIRUS IN PATIENTS WITH A HIGH LEVEL OF

SERUM IgE. *Eur J Immunogenet* 1995; 22: 265-275.

[17] Lorenzo PR 1st null, Kuwabara N, Kondo N, et al. IgE production by B-cells stimulated with interleukin-4 and Epstein-Barr virus in patients with elevated serum IgE levels. *J Investig Allergol Clin Immunol* 1995; 5: 78-81.

[18] Liang Y, Wang P, Zhao M, et al. Demethylation of the FCER1G promoter leads to FcεRI overexpression on monocytes of patients with atopic dermatitis: DNA methylation regulates AD monocyte FcεRI expression. *Allergy* 2012; 67: 424-430.

[19] Novak N. New insights into the mechanism and management of allergic diseases: atopic dermatitis. *Allergy* 2009; 64: 265-275.

[20] Novak N, Allam P, Geiger E, et al. Characterization of monocyte subtypes in the allergic form of atopic eczema/dermatitis syndrome. *Allergy* 2002; 57: 931-935.

[21] Ying S, O'Connor B, Ratoff J, et al. Thymic Stromal Lymphopoietin Expression Is Increased in Asthmatic Airways and Correlates with Expression of Th2-Attracting Chemokines and Disease Severity. *J Immunol* 2005; 174: 8183-8190.

[22] Yoo J, Omori M, Gyarmati D, et al. Spontaneous atopic dermatitis in mice expressing an inducible thymic stromal lymphopoietin transgene specifically in the skin. *Journal of Experimental Medicine* 2005; 202: 541-549.

[23] Millington GW. Epigenetics and dermatological disease. *Pharmacogenomics* 2008; 9: 1835-1850.

[24] Soumelis V, Reche PA, Kanzler H, et al. Human epithelial cells trigger dendritic cell–mediated allergic inflammation by producing TSLP. *Nat Immunol* 2002; 3: 673-680.

[25] Crossno JT, Majka SM, Grazia T, et al. Rosiglitazone promotes development of a novel adipocyte population from bone marrow–derived circulating progenitor cells. *J Clin Invest* 2006; 116: 3220-3228.

[26] Luo Y, Zhou B, Zhao M, et al. Promoter demethylation contributes to TSLP overexpression in skin lesions of patients with atopic dermatitis. *Clin Exp Dermatol* 2014; 39: 48-53.

[27] Wang I-J, Chen S-L, Lu T-P, et al. Prenatal smoke exposure, DNA methylation, and childhood atopic dermatitis. *Clin Exp Allergy* 2013; 43: 535-543.

[28] Cho H-J, Sheen YH, Kang M-J, et al. Prenatal 25-hydroxyvitamin D deficiency affects development of atopic dermatitis via DNA methylation. *Journal of Allergy and Clinical Immunology* 2019; 143: 1215-1218.

[29] Terman JR, Mao T, Pasterkamp RJ, et al. MICALs, a Family of Conserved Flavoprotein Oxidoreductases, Function in Plexin-Mediated Axonal Repulsion. *Cell* 2002; 109: 887-900.

[30] Ba X, Bacsi A, Luo J, et al. 8-Oxoguanine DNA Glycosylase-1 Augments Proinflammatory Gene Expression by Facilitating the Recruitment of Site-Specific Transcription Factors. *JI* 2014; 192: 2384-2394.

[31] Noh Y-H, Lee J, Seo SJ, et al. Promoter DNA methylation contributes to human *β* -defensin-1 deficiency in atopic dermatitis. *Animal Cells and Systems* 2018; 22: 172-177.

[32] The ENCODE Project Consortium. Identification and analysis of functional elements in 1% of the human genome by

the ENCODE pilot project. *Nature* 2007; 447: 799-816.

[33] Han J, Park S-G, Bae J-B, et al. The characteristics of genome-wide DNA methylation in naïve CD4+ T cells of patients with psoriasis or atopic dermatitis. *Biochemical and Biophysical Research Communications* 2012; 422: 157-163.

[34] Libert C, Dejager L, Pinheiro I. The X chromosome in immune functions: when a chromosome makes the difference. *Nat Rev Immunol* 2010; 10: 594-604.

[35] Kaslow DC, Migeon BR. DNA methylation stabilizes X chromosome inactivation in eutherians but not in marsupials: evidence for multistep maintenance of mammalian X dosage compensation. *Proceedings of the National Academy of Sciences* 1987; 84: 6210-6214.

[36] Rodríguez E, Baurecht H, Wahn AF, et al. An Integrated Epigenetic and Transcriptomic Analysis Reveals Distinct Tissue-Specific Patterns of DNA Methylation Associated with Atopic Dermatitis. *Journal of Investigative Dermatology* 2014; 134: 1873-1883.

[37] Olisova OYu, Kochergin NG, Kayumova LN, et al. Skin DNA methylation profile in atopic dermatitis patients: A case–control study. *Exp Dermatol* 2020; 29: 184-189.

[38] Boorgula MP, Taub MA, Rafaels N, et al. Replicated methylation changes associated with eczema herpeticum and allergic response. *Clin Epigenet* 2019; 11: 122.

[39] Liang Y, Chang C, Lu Q. The Genetics and Epigenetics of Atopic Dermatitis—Filaggrin and Other Polymorphisms. *Clinic Rev Allerg Immunol* 2016; 51: 315-328.

[40] Fontenot JD, Rasmussen JP, Williams LM, et al. Regulatory T Cell Lineage Specification by the Forkhead Transcription Factor Foxp3. *Immunity* 2005; 22: 329-341.

[41] Polansky JK, Kretschmer K, Freyer J, et al. DNA methylation controls Foxp3 gene expression. *Eur J Immunol* 2008; 38: 1654-1663.

[42] Hinz D, Bauer M, Röder S, et al. Cord blood Tregs with stable FOXP3 expression are influenced by prenatal environment and associated with atopic dermatitis at the age of one year. *Allergy* 2012; 67: 380-389.

[43] White GP, Watt PM, Holt BJ, et al. Differential Patterns of Methylation of the IFN-γ Promoter at CpG and Non-CpG Sites Underlie Differences in IFN-γ Gene Expression Between Human Neonatal and Adult CD45RO $^-$ T Cells. *J Immunol* 2002; 168: 2820-2827.

[44] Kaminuma O, Kitamura F, Miyatake S, et al. T-box 21 transcription factor is responsible for distorted TH2 differentiation in human peripheral CD4+ T cells. *Journal of Allergy and Clinical Immunology* 2009; 123: 813-823.e3.

[45] Brand S, Teich R, Dicke T, et al. Epigenetic regulation in murine offspring as a novel mechanism for transmaternal asthma protection induced by microbes. *Journal of Allergy and Clinical Immunology* 2011; 128: 618-625.e7.

[46] Makeyev EV, Maniatis T. Multilevel Regulation of Gene Expression by MicroRNAs. *Science* 2008; 319: 1789-1790.

[47] Sonkoly E, Janson P, Majuri M-L, et al. MiR-155 is overexpressed in patients with atopic dermatitis and modulates T-cell proliferative responses by targeting cytotoxic

T lymphocyte–associated antigen 4. *Journal of Allergy and Clinical Immunology* 2010; 126: 581-589.e20.

[48] Herberth G, Bauer M, Gasch M, et al. Maternal and cord blood miR-223 expression associates with prenatal tobacco smoke exposure and low regulatory T-cell numbers. *Journal of Allergy and Clinical Immunology* 2014; 133: 543-550.e4.

Chapter 4

Atmospheric Pollution and Atopic Dermatitis

Gael Ananfack, Mazou Ngou Temgoua and Joel Noutakdie Tochie

Abstract

Atopic dermatitis is a frequent allergic dermatological disorder seen frequently in childhood. Affected patients often have a genetic predisposition and other atopic diseases like asthma, hay fever and allergic rhinitis. There are several triggering factors for atopic dermatitis among which the most recently established one is atmospheric or air pollution. The latter is due to the increased in industrialization in cities with the emission of waste products in the atmosphere as air pollutants. The role played by these pollutants in the pathogenesis of atopic dermatitis still remains largely unclear. This chapter elucidates the relationship between atmospheric pollution and atopic dermatitis.

Keywords: atopic, dermatitis, air, pollution, effects

1. Introduction

Atopic dermatitis (AD) is a chronic inflammatory dermatosis of multifactorial aetiologies. It is a common disease that frequently occurs in childhood. A rising prevalence rate of AD over the past six decades has been reported to be mainly due to several environmental factors [1, 2]. In the interplay between the interactions predisposing genes, environmental factors, impaired skin barrier integrity, skin microbiota, and immune deregulation are at the core of the pathogenesis of AD [3]. Established risk factors for AD include a regular diet rich in fresh fruits and fish during pregnancy leading to AD in offspring of these women during childhood. Avoiding such a diet by pregnant women has been demonstrated to reduce both the prevalence and incidence of AD in children and adolescents [4–6]. Furthermore, it has been reported that a family history of asthma, hay fever, or eczema is associated with AD in childhood and this risk increases if both parents have eczema [7]. Persons of similar racial and genetic background are at an increased risk of AD in metropolitan areas compared with countryside individuals [8]. Urbanization and industrialization often occur together. Industrialization in urban areas is often associated with atmospheric or air pollution which can be mild to severe depending on the degree of industries startups in the town or city concerned. The air pollution stemming from these industries has recently been positively correlated to the development of AD. However, the relationship between atmospheric or air pollution and AD still largely remains to be elucidated. With the several advancements made in industrialization, there is emerging of some chronic diseases which share the same pathophysiological mechanisms with AD. Thus it is important to evaluate the contribution of atmospheric pollution in the growing burden of AD.

2. Atmospheric or air pollution and chronic inflammatory diseases

Although air pollution is well known to be harmful to the lung and airways, it can also damage most other organ systems of the body. Pollution affects the immune system and is associated with allergic rhinitis, hypersensitivity disorders, and autoimmune diseases. The lung has a large surface area that comes into contact with a myriad of antigens. It sensitization effect and antigen-presenting system are quite efficacious and this consequently makes individuals susceptible to autoimmune diseases. The pollution of air markedly contributes to illnesses such as systemic lupus erythematosus and rheumatoid arthritis [9]. A Canadian study found increased odds of having a diagnosis of a rheumatic disease following an increased exposure to ambient particulate matter with an aerodynamic diameter < 2.5 mm ($PM_{2.5}$) exposure [10]. Air pollutants have also been described to trigger or exacerbate diseases like juvenile idiopathic arthritis, but the impaired autoimmunity related to exposure to air pollution has largely been understudied. Inflammation in the bloodstream in response to air pollutants has been found to cause systemic vascular (including cerebral vascular) dysfunctions. Studies on animals observed that inhaled ultrafine particles from the atmosphere into the nostrils then get in contact with the neighbouring olfactory nerve and later to the central nervous system, particularly to the brain leading to inflammatory and oxidative stress responses [11]. In all the organs that are affected by air pollution, the skin is one of the most frequently involved leading to atopic skin disease.

3. Atmospheric or air pollution and atopic dermatitis

3.1 Evidence

Since almost one-third of patients with AD develop this skin disorder within their first year of life, it may be important to consider the impact of prenatal exposure to air pollution. In a study published almost a decade ago and involving 469 pregnant women, prenatal exposure to fine air pollutants (fine air particulate matter—$PM_{2.5}$) with subsequent postnatal exposure to the same air pollutants and cigarette smoke had their children followed up every three months for a year [12]. The prevalence of AD during the first year of life increased by two-fold [12]. Likewise, a Swedish study showed an association between AD and lower ventilation in the houses, in particular, in the child's bedrooms [13]. Furthermore, a German study found an association between indoor renovation activities (painting, furniture, and floor covering) and the antenatal period, infantile period and early childhood and lifetime prevalence of AD, likely in connection with high levels of volatile organic compounds (VOCs) [14]. More still, a study of 317,926 Taiwanese children found a significant positive association between traffic-related air pollutants such as carbon monoxide, nitrogen oxides and AD in both sexes [15]. In the same vein, a study conducted on 4907 French children found associations of both history and lifetime of AD with urban air pollutants such as NOx, CO, NO_2, PM10, and benzene pollutants [16].

A USA population-based study found the prevalence of childhood AD to be associated with mean annual NO_2, sulfur dioxide (SO_2), and sulfur trioxide (SO_3) [17]. A German birth cohort study found that the rates of AD in the first children aged one to six years old was positively correlated with the degree of home proximity to motorable roads [18]. Also, the distance from home to the closest road was used as the main indicator of air pollution due to road traffics. The highest odds of AD occurred in children <50 m from the main road [18]. The authors postulated that residents living closer to heavy traffic are exposed to both higher amounts of and more toxic air pollutants that are freshly emitted from vehicles moving on these roads. Two longitudinal studies assessed the relationship between outdoor pollution and childhood AD symptom severity. A South Korean study of 41 children aged 8–12 years collected symptom diaries for 67 days and found significant associations between pruritus severity and daily ambient air particulate matter concentrations [19]. A longer-term study of 22 Korean children using symptom diaries for 18 months also found associations of AD symptoms with levels of outdoor air pollutants [20]. From the aforementioned data, it is clear that outdoor and indoor air pollution can cause, trigger and/or exacerbate AD.

3.2 Pathophysiology

As an allergic disease, the triggers of AD may originate from indoor and/or outdoor environmental factors and can interact with the skin by binding to the stratum corneum, becoming metabolized, or even penetrating the epidermis and entering systemic circulation through dermal capillaries [21]. The biomechanical effect of particulate matter is not entirely clear. It contains a myriad of toxic substances such as tobacco and alloy smoke, polycyclic aromatic hydrocarbons, organic compounds, nitrates, sulphates and metals. These particulates have the capacity to cross through the skin, the respiratory tract and blood placental barrier. They also have a slow index of sedimentation. Hence, they remain as air suspension over a longtime where they have dust mites and pollen 'carrier' effects due to their protein linking ability. When pregnant women are exposed to polycyclic hydrocarbons, this has several adverse effects to the foetas. These negative foetal effects include the formation of free radicals, activation of apoptosis, and the production of IgE and cytokines. Postnatal exposure to air pollutants increases the effects of prenatal exposure and has been implicated in lesions to the skin barrier, with a resulting inflammatory process [12, 22, 23]. There are likely multiple mechanisms for the harmful effects of different air pollutants. A study of skin biopsies from 75 AD patients found an association between severe AD and reactive oxygen species-related damage. This finding is in favour of the hypothesis that reactive oxygen species originating from environmental exposures cause oxidative stress damage to proteins in the stratum corneum [24]. Even short-term exposure to NO_2 or volatile organic compounds (VOC) caused significantly increased trans-epidermal water loss (TEWL) in both healthy individuals and those with AD [23, 25]. VOC may also contribute to T helper 2 (Th-2) polarization, suggesting potentially direct effects of pollutants on the immune system [26].

4. Public health implications

Air pollution is a public health problem today. Its ill-health effects are increasing worldwide. Assessing these effects may be difficult because the source of air pollution varies between communities and household situations. Governments should, therefore, put in place measures to reduce environmental air pollution in the aforementioned high-risk areas (e.g. those living close to the roadside) and people-centered measures such as facemasks which can reduce inhaled particulates. For instance, wearing personal respirators such as facemasks while being active in central Beijing reduced the blood pressure (BP) and heart rate variability, and markers associated with cardiovascular morbidity [27]. The beneficial effects of the use of personal respirators on cardiovascular parameters markers were almost immediate and lasted during the entire exposure time [28]. Air purifiers also reduce air particulate matters. Air purification for just 48 hours significantly decreased $PM_{2.5}$ and reduced circulating inflammatory and thrombogenic biomarkers as well as systolic and diastolic BPs.

5. Conclusion

Atopic dermatitis is a growing disease; the risk factors are numerous and include air pollution. Air pollutants act by several mechanisms including the synthesis of reactive oxygen species which will cause a weakening of the skin barrier and thus exposes individuals to various degrees of atopic dermatitis. The increasing urbanization and development of countries that increase air pollution will probably aggravate this disease. Air pollution has a proven effect on the burden of AD. This should sensitize the general population especially AD patients and public health authorities in particular about the impact of air pollution on pollution health, especially dermatology health.

Author details

Gael Ananfack[1], Mazou Ngou Temgoua[1] and Joel Noutakdie Tochie[2,3,4*]

1 Department of Internal Medicine and Subspecialties, Faculty of Medicine and Biomedical Sciences, University of Yaoundé I, Yaoundé, Cameroon

2 Department of Anesthesiology and Critical Care Medicine, Faculty of Medicine and Biomedical Sciences, University of Yaoundé I, Yaoundé, Cameroon

3 Human Research Education and Networking, Yaoundé, Cameroon

4 Faculty of Medicine and Biomedical Sciences, Yaoundé, University of Yaoundé I, Cameroon

*Address all correspondence to: joeltochie@gmail.com

References

[1] Kantor R, Silverberg JI. Environmental risk factors and their role in the management of atopic dermatitis. Expert Review of Clinical Immunology. 2017;**13**(1):15-26

[2] Mohammad KAA, Ali MB, Buddenkotte J, Mounir M, Gerber R, Mohamed HA, et al. Understanding the burden of atopic dermatitis in Africa and the Middle East. Dermatol Ther (Heidelb). 2019;**9**:223-241

[3] Manousaki D, Paternoster L, Standl M, Mo_att MF, Farrall M, Bouzigon E, et al. Vitamin D levels and susceptibility to asthma, elevated immunoglobulin E levels, and atopic dermatitis: A Mendelian randomization study. PLoS Medicine. 2017;**14**:e1002294

[4] Romieu I, Torrent M, Garcia-Esteban R, Ferrer C, Ribas-Fitó N, Antó JM, et al. Maternal fish intake during pregnancy and atopy and asthma in infancy. Clinical and Experimental Allergy. 2007;**37**:518-525

[5] Leermakers ETM, der Voort S-VAMM, Heppe DHM, de Jongste JC, Moll HA, Franco OH, et al. Maternal fish consumption during pregnancy and risks of wheezing and eczema in childhood: The generation R study. European Journal of Clinical Nutrition. 2013;**67**:353-359

[6] Willers SM, Devereux G, Craig LCA, McNeill G, Wijga AH, El-Magd AW, et al. Maternal food consumption during pregnancy and asthma, respiratory and atopic symptoms in 5-year-old children. Thorax. 2007;**62**:773-779

[7] Apfelbacher CJ, Diepgen TL, Schmitt J. Determinants of eczema: Population-based cross-sectional study in Germany. Allergy. 2011;**66**:206-213

[8] Hugg TR, Ruotsalainen MS, Pushkarev JJ, Jaakkola JV. Comparison of allergic diseases, symptoms and respiratory infections between Finnish and Russian school children. European Journal of Epidemiology. 2008;**23**(2):123-133

[9] Farhat SC, Silva CA, Orione MA, Campos LM, Sallum AM, Braga AL. Air pollution in autoimmune rheumatic diseases: A review. Autoimmunity Reviews 2011;11(1):14-21

[10] Bernatsky S, Smargiassi A, Barnabe C, et al. Fine particulate air pollution and systemic autoimmune rheumatic disease in two Canadian provinces. Environmental Research. 2016;**146**:85-91

[11] Elder A, Gelein R, Silva V, et al. Translocation of inhaled ultrafine manganese oxide particles to the central nervous system. Environmental Health Perspectives. 2006;**114**(8):1172-1178

[12] Jedrychowski W, Perera F, Maugeri U, et al. Effects of prenatal and perinatal exposure to fine air pollutants and maternal fish consumption on the occurrence of infantile eczema. International Archives of Allergy and Immunology. 2011;**155**(3):275-281

[13] Bornehag CG, Sundell J, Hagerhed-Engman L, Sigsgaard T. Association between ventilation rates in 390 Swedish homes and allergic symptoms in children. Indoor Air. 2005;**15**(4):275-280

[14] Herbarth OG, Fritz JM, Richter RM, Roder S, Schlink U. Association between indoor renovation activities and eczema in early childhood. International Journal of Hygiene and Environmental Health. 2006;**209**(3):241-247

[15] Lee Y-L, Su H-J, Sheu H-M, et al. Traffic-related air pollution, climate, and prevalence of eczema in Taiwanese school children. The Journal of Investigative Dermatology. 2008;**128**:2412-2420

[16] Pénard-Morand C, Raherison C, Charpin D, et al. Long-term exposure to close-proximity air pollution and asthma and allergies in urban children. The European Respiratory Journal. 2010;**36**:33-40

[17] Kathuria P, Silverberg JI. Association between small particle air pollution, climate and childhood eczema prevalence and severity: A US population-based study. Pediatric Allergy and Immunology. 2016;**27**(5):478-485

[18] Morgenstern V, Zutavern A, Cyrys J, et al. Atopic diseases, allergic sensitization, and exposure to traffic-related air pollution in children. American Journal of Respiratory and Critical Care Medicine. 2008;**177**:1331-1337

[19] Song S, Lee K, Lee Y-M, et al. Acute health effects of urban fine and ultrafine particles on children with atopic dermatitis. Environmental Research. 2011;**111**:394-399

[20] Kim J, Kim E-H, Oh I, et al. Symptoms of atopic dermatitis are influenced by outdoor air pollution. The Journal of Allergy and Clinical Immunology. 2013;**132**:495-498. e491

[21] Ahn K. The role of air pollutants in atopic dermatitis. The Journal of Allergy and Clinical Immunology. 2014;**134**(5):993-999

[22] KimJ KE-H, Oh I, et al. Symptoms of atopic dermatitis are influenced by outdoor air pollution. The Journal of Allergy and Clinical Immunology. 2013;**132**(2):495-497

[23] Huss-Marp J, Eberlein-Konig B, Breuer K, et al. Influence of short-term exposure to airborne Der p 1 and volatile organic compounds on skin barrier function and dermal blood flow in patients with atopic eczema and healthy individuals. Clinical & Experimental Allergy. 2006;**36**(3):338-345

[24] Niwa Y, Sumi H, Kawahira K, et al. Protein oxidative damage in the stratum corneum: Evidence for a link between environmental oxidants and the changing prevalence and nature of atopic dermatitis in Japan. The British Journal of Dermatology. 2003;**149**(248):254

[25] Eberlein-König B, Przybilla B, Kühnl P, et al. Influence of airborne nitrogen dioxide or formaldehyde on parameters of skin function and cellular activation in patients with atopic eczema and control subjects. The Journal of Allergy and Clinical Immunology. 1998;**101**:141-143

[26] Lehmann I, Rehwagen M, Diez U, et al. Enhanced in vivo IgE production and T cell polarization toward the type 2 phenotype in association with indoor exposure to VOC: Results of the LARS study. International Journal of Hygiene and Environmental Health. 2001;**204**:211-221

[27] Langrish JP, Mills NL, Chan JK, et al. Beneficial cardiovascular effects of reducing exposure to particulate air pollution with a simple facemask. Particle and Fibre Toxicology. 2009;**6**:8

[28] Yang X, Jia X, Dong W, et al. Cardiovascular benefits of reducing personal exposure to traffic-related noise and particulate air pollution: A randomized crossover study in the Beijing subway system. Indoor Air. DOI: 10.1111/ina.12485. [Accessed: 03 June 2020]

Chapter 5

Atopic Dermatitis in Adults: Epidemiology, Risk Factors, Pathogenesis, Clinical Features, and Management

Olumayowa Abimbola Oninla, Ayesha Omolara Akinkugbe, Bolaji Ibiesa Otike-Odibi, Mufutau Muphy Oripelaye and Fatai Olatunde Olanrewaju

Abstract

Atopic dermatitis (AD) is an itchy chronic relapsing inflammatory skin condition mostly affecting children than adults. Eczematous conditions are common worldwide with increase in the prevalence in both developed and developing countries. AD in adults is of two types – the first type starts as AD in childhood and gradually progresses to adulthood (Persistent AD) and the second type results from AD developing in adulthood (Adult-onset AD). The article reviews and discusses this condition in adults considering the epidemiology, risk factors, pathogenesis, diagnostic criteria, and management of this condition.

Keywords: Atopic dermatitis, Adult, Adult-onset Atopic dermatitis, Eczema

1. Introduction

Atopic dermatitis (AD) is an itchy chronic relapsing inflammatory skin condition mostly affecting children than adults with atopy. Atopy was derived from the Greek word "atopos" by Coca and Cooke in 1923 for the grouping of asthma, hay fever and asthma. [1] In an article by Kanwar, atopic dermatitis (AD) or atopic eczema was defined as "an itchy, inflammatory skin condition characterized by poorly defined erythema with edema, vesicles, and weeping in the acute stage and skin thickening (lichenification) in the chronic stage," [2] and in the year 2000, Bannister and Freeman originated the term adult-onset atopic dermatitis for the condition in adulthood. [3] AD usually occur as a continuum of childhood AD but few cases start in adulthood, hence, the term - Adult onset AD. AD in adults is of two types – the first type occurs as AD in childhood and progresses to adulthood condition (Persistent AD) while the second type results from AD developing in adulthood (Adult-onset AD). Eczema in adults usually runs a prolong course impairing quality of life, relationships and sex life, and occupation. [4]

Atopy refers to "the genetic tendency to develop allergic diseases such as allergic rhinitis, asthma and atopic dermatitis (eczema). Atopy is typically associated with heightened immune responses to common allergens, especially inhaled allergens and food allergens." [5] Rang et al. defined atopy as 'a familial hypersensitivity of the skin and the mucosa to environmental substances, associated with increased production of immunoglobulin E (IgE) or altered pharmacologic reactivity.' [6] The ETFAD/EADV Eczema task force consensus 2020 defines atopy as the 'familial tendency to develop Th2 responses against common environmental antigens. [7]

The definition by ETFAD/EADV encompasses both subtypes of atopy – the extrinsic (IgE-associated) subtype, and the intrinsic (non-IgE-associated) subtype. Most AD affected persons have atopic diathesis. The Japanese Dermatological Association defines atopic diathesis as: (1) Personal or family history (asthma, allergic rhinitis and/or conjunctivitis, and atopic dermatitis), and/or (2) Predisposition to overproduction of immunoglobulin E (IgE) antibodies. [8] The Japanese Dermatological Association criteria is based on three clinical features that must be present for diagnosis of AD: (1) pruritus, (2) exanthematous features and their distribution, and (3) chronically relapsing course.

2. Etiology

The increasing number of adult AD cases in recent years has elicited interest in determining factors causing and modifying the disease in adults. Susceptibility to AD is attributable to both genetic and environmental causes. [9] The study by Thomsen et al., showed that AD susceptibility and incidence are mainly due to genetics with 82% cases of AD associated with genes and 18% associated with nonshared environmental factors. [9] A monozyotic twin of an affected person has a sevenfold risk of developing AD compared with a threefold increased risk in dizygotic twin. [9]

Intrinsic IgE-mediated allergic inflammation may play an important role in the pathobiology of elderly AD, similar to other age groups of AD. [10] About 5–15% of cases have intrinsic non-IgE-allergic eczema. [4] Most of the adult AD patients have sensitivity to aeroallergens such as cat epithet, dog epithel and housedusthouse dust mites [11] while common food allergies affect only few. [4] There is a high incidence of contact sensitization to environmental allergens such as nickel (in metals), thiomersal (in eyedrops), fragrance mix (in cosmetics) and lanalcolum (in cosmetics) in adult AD. [11] An increased occurrence of occupational allergic and irritant contact dermatitis among adult AD cases have also been observed. [4] Immunoglobulin E-mediated tests, atopy patch tests (APT), epicutaneous tests (ET), in vitro allergy and Prick tests are usually positive on contact with environmental allergens and to aero allergens. [11]. Pollens are associated with seasonal relapse of AD.

There is specific immediate and delayed sensibilization to Malassezia sympodialis in both intrinsic and extrinsic AD in adults. High rates of sensitization to Dermatophagoides farinae and/or Dermatophagoides pteronyssinus have been documented in patients with extrinsic allergy. House door mite (HDM) refers to a large number of dust dwelling mites including the American HDM, Dermatophagoides farinae Hughes, and the European HDM, Dermatophagoides pteronyssinus. HDM is a common household aeroallergen known to cause asthma, allergic rhinitis and AD. The indoor level of HDM is associated with the severity of skin lesions. [12]

The proportion of contact sensitization to environmental allergens in the 34 adult atopic patients was remarkable (14 of 34, 41%). Out of the verified contact allergens, nickel, fragrance mix, thimerosal and lanalcolum proved to be relevant. House dust mite and cat epithel proved to be the most common relevant aeroallergens. *D. pteronyssinus* and D. farinae sensibilization was high, particularly in patients with severe skin symptoms on the face, eyelids and hands. Pollens should be considered in patients with seasonal relapse of AD. Sensitization to animal epithel was usually indicated by the flare-up of skin symptoms upon contact with animals. The relevance of the eliciting effects of sensitization could easily be supported in most cases by the medical history and the distribution of skin symptoms. In some adult AD patients with long-lasting AD, the relevance of triggering factors is hard to determine.

The intrinsic (non-IgE-allergic) eczema subtype affects 5–15% of cases. Classical food allergy has a low importance, although non-IgE-mediated and pseudoallergic reactions can cause eczema. Sensitivity to aeroallergens, especially dust mite, is demonstrated in the majority of adult AD patients, including elderly adults, by immunoglobulin E-mediated tests and/or atopy patch tests. Occupational allergic and irritant contact dermatitis is increased. In adults, as in children, *Staphylococcus aureus* colonization is very high, whereas adult skin is more heavily colonized with Malassezia yeasts. Immediate and delayed sensitization to Malassezia sympodialis is specific for intrinsic and extrinsic AD, occurring especially in head-and-neck eczema. [4]

In the study by Pónyai et al., [11] atopy patch and epicutaneous tests (APT, ET), which were supplemented by in vitro allergy and Prick tests – sensibilization was evaluated by the comparison of in vivo and in vitro test results, medical history and skin symptoms. The incidence of contact sensitization to environmental allergens was remarkable: 13 of the EG, 1 of the IG (14 of 34, 41%) The allergens causing positivity were nickel (6 of 13), thiomersal (3 of 13), mercury-amidochlorate (3 of 13), mercury-chloride (2 of 13), iodine chlorhyrdoxyquin (1 of 13), lanalcolum (1 of 13) and fragrance mix (1 of 13). Among the detected allergens, the following were relevant: lanalcolum (1 of 13: cosmetics), fragrance mix (1 of 13: cosmetics), nickel (1 of 13: metal objects), thiomersal (1 of 13: eyedrops).

3. Epidemiology

Atopic dermatitis often develops in infancy with *about* 75% occurring at less than 6 months and 90% before 5 years with about 60–70% resolving in the early teenage years. [1] AD is manly a disease of children with prevalence of 10–20% in children in developed countries. [13] A prevalent rate of 6% was found among children by Oninla et al. [14] at a dermatology centre while Ayanlowo et al. [15] documented a prevalence of 15% at another dermatology centre in Nigeria, a developing country.

Adult AD prevalence is 1–3% of adults world-wide. [4] Approximately 40% of childhood AD persist till adulthood. [16] Adult-onset AD was reported by 1 out of 4 adults with AD. [17] Variable age of onset of adult AD from 18 to 71 years has been reported. [2] About 9% of the cases seen at a contact dermatitis clinic had AD with first onset at 20 years and above while an additional 8% had both adult-onset AD and contact dermatitis. [18] An incidence rate of 18% was reported among adults presenting at a contact dermatitis clinic in a study by the Postgraduate Institute of Medical Education and Research (PGIMER), Chandigarh. A female preponderance was found in adult AD in some studies though no gender predilection was reported in children. [16, 18]

4. Risk factors

Atopic dermatitis runs a chronic course with acute exacerbations due to triggers such as exposure to allergens (commonly pollens), skin irritants (for example woolen fabrics, exfoliating soaps, and detergents), stress conditions, skin dryness, dry weather conditions, skin infections and food such as peanuts, gluten, eggs, soy, dairy products and alcohol. [17] Persistence of atopic dermatitis till adulthood was associated with early onset AD, childhood allergic rhinitis, hand eczema, allergic contact dermatitis and increased specific IgE to *Malassezia furfur*. [19]

5. Pathogenesis

Various studies reported AD as a disease resulting from a complex interplay of genetic factors, immunologic mechanisms, biochemical factors, environmental triggers, and pharmacologic factors. [20–24] Sehra et al., [24] described the pathogenesis of this disease and stated that it should translate to treatment strategies. In the review by Leung, [20] AD was initially considered as a disease mediated by a bone-marrow derived cell. This was based on the report that a bone marrow transplant from an AD donor in positive immediate skin tests and symptoms of atopy in the recipient. Also, patients with primary T cell immunodeficiency disorders were found to have elevated serum IgE levels, eosinophilia, and skin lesions of AD. Recently, Leung along with other researchers' reported that AD occurs as a complex interplay of immunologic, microbial, and epithelial interactions. [25]

Recent evidence also revealed that the underlying pathogenesis of AD has shifted from focusing primarily on generalized immune system abnormalities in Th1/Th2 cells to a complex interplay between primary epithelial barrier defect in skin membrane (possibly a genetic defect) and dysregulation of immunological mechanisms involving specific signaling pathways. [25, 26] These abnormalities lead to membrane barrier defects resulting in increased transepidermal water loss (TEWL) and increased allergen exposure as well as immunologic alteration toward atopy. [27]

The exact pathogenesis remains unclear and the underlying mechanism that is well known in the disease development and progression has been atopy. Children with early onset AD often develop allergies to common environmental or food allergens or infective agent [28] with positive skin prick test (SPT) or elevated antigen-specific serum immunoglobulin E (IgE). This type of AD where specific IgE plays a central role in AD is known as Extrinsic AD. The severity of AD has been found to correlate directly with the number of SPT and/or levels of antigen-specific IgE. [29] Extrinsic form accounts for about 45–75% of AD cases. [24]

Although total Ig E elevation is mostly seen in many AD individuals, other factors also modulate the pathophysiology of AD giving rise to the non-atopic or non-T-2 inflammation form of the disease. These are: genetic factors, age, gender, maternal history of atopy, [24] ethnicity, [30] socioeconomic status, [31] environmental factors, and early daycare attendance. [24] The intrinsic form might also affect as many as two thirds of AD individuals. [32]

5.1 Pathogenic mechanisms

5.1.1 Epidermal barrier dysfunction

A strong family history has been reported in 40–60% of AD patients with filaggrin (FLG) null mutation in 20–30%. [33, 34] Genetic mutations involving the epidermal differentiation complex (EDC) gene on chromosome 1q21 impairs epidermal differentiation resulting in stratum corneum barrier dysfunction. [35] The nonsense mutations occur in the EDC gene encoding FLG which is also implicated in asthma associated with AD. [36–38] The gene codes for profilaggrin, a large precursor protein molecule which is subsequently hydrolyzed to ten to twelve units of FLG. [39]

Palmer et al., reported two independent loss-of-function genetic variants - R510X and 2282del4 - mutations of the skin barrier gene encoding filaggrin (FLG) as very strong predisposing factors. [38] FLG, a filament aggregating protein, binds keratin intermediate fibers to the envelope of the stratum corneum cells and facilitates terminal differentiation of the epidermis. [38] Therefore, filaggrin is needed for the formation of skin barrier to maintain hydration and provide protection from environmental insults and infective agents. [40, 41] Recent studies have linked genetic FLG mutations to Th2 mediated AD and not non-Th2 inflammation AD giving rise to suggestions that skin barrier defect underlies the development of secondary allergic symptoms and respiratory atopy. [24] The degree of membrane disruption directly correlates with the severity of AD. [42]

The study by Pellerin et al. showed that the stratum corneum of lesional skin as well as the clinically nonlesional skin of adults AD patients has reduced expression of FLG and FLG-like proteins. [43] This was found to be as a result of nonsense mutations, proinflammatory cytokines and some defects in the proFLG processing. The study concluded that skin inflammation contributing to the AD-related epidermal barrier dysfunction is by downregulation of FLG and FLG-like proteins. FLG mutation has been identified as the most common genetic factor associated with AD and present in 15–50%. [44] However, 40% of FLG mutant gene carrier do not have AD. [38]

The epithelium in AD also have decreased barrier-stabilizing proteins such as loricrin (LOR), involucrin (IVL), and proline rich particles. [44] Tumor necrosis factor-alpha and interleukin (IL)-4 result in downregulation of LOR and filaggrin (FLG). [29, 45] In AD lesional skin, lipid synthesis is reduced [46] due to increased expression of enzyme stearoyl-CoA desaturase leading to increased unsaturated fatty acids and abnormal keratinization. [47] Th2 cytokines and IFN-γ also reduces long-chain free fatty acids (FFA) and ester linked-hydroxy (EO) ceramides in the skin membrane. [48, 49]

Many researchers have reported that defective skin barrier particularly in the epidermis preludes the pathologies seen in AD development mainly in the following ways: [26, 50–52].

- Defects in epidermal proteins such as FLG, keratins, transglutaminases, loricrin, involucrin reduces skin hydration and inflammatory thresholds while increasing skin pH, inflammatory cytokines, and allergen and microbes permeability. [26]

- Reduction in claudins increases transepidermal water loss (TEWL), reduces hydration, and allows allergens and microorganisms invasion. [53]

- Decreased long-chain FFA and ceramides increases TEWL and infections. [26]

- Decreased cathelicidin and human β-defensins increase microbial infections (mostly *Staph. aureus*) and pro-inflammatory cytokines. [26]

5.1.2 Immune system dysregulation

Polymorphisms of genes in the Th2 signaling pathway particularly cytokine receptors (IL-4R and IL-13R) are associated with immune dysfunction in AD. [54–57] Also implicated are genes transcribing for IL-31 and IL-33, thymic stromal lymphopoietin (TSLP) and its receptors (IL-7R and TSLPR), interferon regulatory factor 2, signal transducer and activator of transcription (STAT) 6, Toll-like receptor 2, and high-affinity IgE receptor (FcRI), [26, 54, 56, 58–60] vitamin D receptor and cytochrome P450 (CYP27A1 variant involved in D3 metabolism). [61, 62] Environmental factors (mostly allergens, microorganisms, smoke, and chemical irritants) also cause modifications in DNA resulting in epidermal and genetic changes (epigenetic changes) without changing the DNA sequence of the corneocytes. [56]

Of recent, the skin epithelium was found to produce IL-25, IL-33, and/or TSLP (in response to extracellular molecules such as parasites and allergens) which activates skin group 2 innate lymphoid cells (ILC2). ILC2 produces IL-5, IL-9 and IL-13 which are Type 2 cytokines. [63] The T_H2 cytokines (IL-4, IL-13, IL-31) and T_H22 cytokine (IL-22) are believed to play roles in the overall pathogenesis of atopic dermatitis but mostly acute AD (**Figure 1**). [64–66]

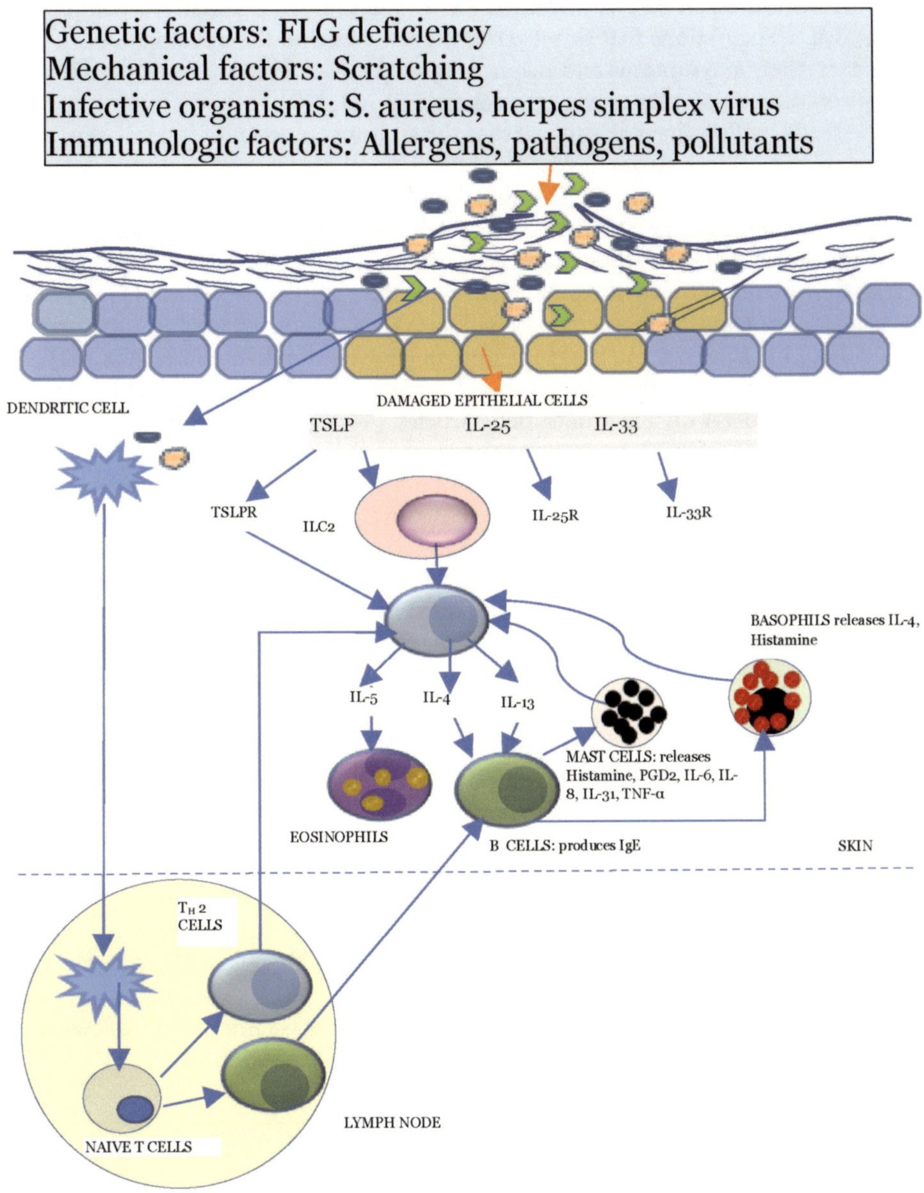

Figure 1.

Pathogenesis of atopic dermatitis. Damage to the skin barrier allows penetration of the skin by allergens, environmental factors and infective organisms activating the skin antigen-presenting cells (APCs). The APCs migrate to lymph nodes and stimulate naive T cells differentiation into TH2 cells and B lymphocytes. Damaged epithelial cells releases TSLP, TNF-α and IFN-γ and other TH2 cytokines (mostly IL-25 and IL-33) which induces mostly TH2 inflammation and subsequently keratinocyte apoptosis.TH2, T helper 2 cells; ILC2, innate lymphoid cell; TSLP, thymic stromal lymphopoietin; TSLPR, thymic stromal lymphopoietin receptor. Cited from reference [100].

IL-4 is primarily produced by mast cells, Th2 cells, oesinophils and basophils. [67] IL-4 stimulates both the humoral and innate immunity. It reduces the expression epidermal differentiation complex (EDC) genes which regulates keratinocytes function. It activates B cell production which ingests antigens and presents them as major histocompatibility complex (MHC) II molecules to which T cells bind leading to cytokine production and signals to other phagocytes. The T cells further stimulate these activated B cells and differentiation into plasma cells leading to antibody production. IL-4 enhances the development of Th2 cells, suppresses the formation of major terminal differentiation proteins by downregulating the encoding genes for FLG, LOR, and IVL, increases fibronectin, and increases adhesion of *S. aureus* to the skin. [64, 68–71]

IL-13 acts similarly to IL-4 and these two are the most frequently produced cytokines by Th2 cells. IL-13 promotes tissue inflammation by inducing cellular migration (CD4+ T-cells, mast cells, eosinophils, and macrophages) to the dermis. [68, 71] Both IL-4 and IL-13 hinders keratinocyte differentiation resulting in membrane barrier dysfunction and increase periostin expression stimulating skin remodeling in chronic AD. [72, 73] They induce cytokines, epidermal dysfunction, suppress antimicrobial peptides (AMP), and stimulates allergic nflammation. [64, 74] Another study by Howell et al., [74] showed that filaggrin gene expression by keratinocytes stimulated by IL-4 and IL-13 was significantly reduced when compared with normal skin. [75]

IL-5 is produced by Th2, eosinophils and mast cells though eosinophils are the primary IL-5Rα-expressing cells. It functions as an eosinophil colony-stimulating factor, B-cells growth factor and increases immunoglobulin secretion – mostly IgA. [68, 76] IL-31, a cytokine mainly produced by CD4+ Th2 cells is a potent mediator of inflammation. [77] Monocytes, epithelial cells, and T cells have the receptor – IL-31R, on their cell membrane. [77] IL-31R induces and potentiates pruritus in AD [76, 78] by production of natriuretic peptide in the brain and chemokine release from keratinocytes. [79]

According to Rebane et al., IFN-γ is the characteristic cytokine induced by Th1 cells. [80] In acute AD, immunoglobulin G (IgG) inhibits the production of IFN-γ. [81] Interferon-gamma is secreted predominantly by activated lymphocytes such as CD4 T helper type 1 (Th1) cells and CD8 cytotoxic T cells. [82] Other cells producing IFN-γ are natural killer (NK) cells, B cells and antigen-presenting cells (APCs) – macrophages, and these cells aggregate in the skin during inflammatory reactions and infections. [83] Werfel et al., reported that CD8 T cells are part of the early cellular response in AD. [84] Higher CD8 IL-13+ 1CLA1 frequencies were seen in adults compared with children with AD. [85] CD8 T cells constitute 15% of allergen-specific T cells in the skin. [86] These cells stimulates the production of interferon-γ (IFN-γ), IL-13, and IL-22. [87–89] It was also reported that IFN-γ upregulated 3 apoptosis-related genes (*NOD2, DUSP1,* and *ADM*) and stimulates the overexpression of 8 genes (*CCDC109B, CCL5, CCL8, IFI35, LYN, RAB31, IFITM1,* and *IFITM2*) in keratinocytes of lesional skin.

TH17-associated molecules (IL-17A, peptidase inhibitor 3/elafin, and CCL20) are consistently upregulated in both patients with acute and chronic AD. IL-17 production is higher in intrinsic AD, and severe AD. [90] It reduces FLG and INV while stimulating antimicrobial peptide human beta-defensin 2 (HBD-2) in keratinocytes. [91, 92]

Apart from elevated IgE levels and eosinophilia, Leung reported that the peripheral blood has the following immunologic responses: [20].

- Increased basophil spontaneous histamine release
- Decreased CD8 suppressor/cytotoxic number and function

- Increased expression of CD23 on mononuclear cells
- Chronic macrophage activation, increased GM-CSF, prostaglandin E2, and IL-10
- Expansion of IL-4– and IL-5–secreting Th2-type cells
- Decreased numbers of IFN-γ–secreting Th1-type cells
- Increased serum sIL-2 receptor levels
- Increased serum eosinophil cationic protein levels
- Increased soluble E-selectin levels
- Increased soluble vascular cell adhesion molecule-1 levels
- Increased soluble intercellular adhesion molecule-1 levels

These immunologic changes underlies the skin inflammatory process in AD.

The cellular and cytokines infiltrates in the skin depends on the duration of the lesion. Cellular infiltrates particularly T cells occur as an immune response in AD patients. T lymphocytes are moderately increased in the dermal layer of nonlesional skin with marked increase in acutely inflamed areas and acute flares of chronic lesions resulting in epidermal cell apoptosis and spongiosis. Nonlesional skin has no eosinophils and macrophages, and cytokines seen are IL_4, IL-13 and IL_16 [20, 80] In acute lesional skin, cellular infiltrates consists of mostly T-cells, moderate amount of inflammatory dendritic cells (IDCs) mostly Langerhans cells, eosinophils, macrophages, IL-4, IL-13, IL-5, IL-22, IL-16, IL-31 and Granulocyte-macrophage colony-stimulating factor (GM-CSF). (20). Chronic lesional skin has mostly eosinophils and macrophages with moderate number of T cells, GM-CSF, and cytokines type are IL-4/13, IL-5, IL-12, IL-16, IL-31 and Interferon-γ. (20).

a. Acute Dermatitis: According to Grittler, AD is currently considered a biphasic disease depending on the type of cellular immune response to numerous environmental antigens and infections. [64] An initial phase of acute disease characterized by predominantly Th2 cells, as well as Th_H22 and few eosinophils progresses to a chronic disease and a switch to mostly Th1 cells, and Th17 cells. Th2 lymphocytes are the most predominant cells in all AD phenotypes, and play a key role in all allergic inflammation. [40, 93] Infiltration by Th2 cells are more in the acute phase than other phenotypes. These cells are targeted in immunotherapy for precision medicine. [94, 95]

b. Chronic Dermatitis: Allergen specific T-cell clone (TCC) from spontaneous chronic lesional skin of AD patients was found different from the TCC isolated from inhalant allergen patch test lesions. [86] These TCC are allergen-nonspecific cells that produce IFN-γ and the chronic changes seen in the skin and were found to be Th1 cells. [84] Many other studies also reported that Th1 cells increases in the lesions in chronic AD from an initial Th2 polarization. [96–98]

The Janus kinase-signal transducer and activator of transcription (JAK/STAT) pathway acts downstream of more than 50 cytokines. [99] It is central to

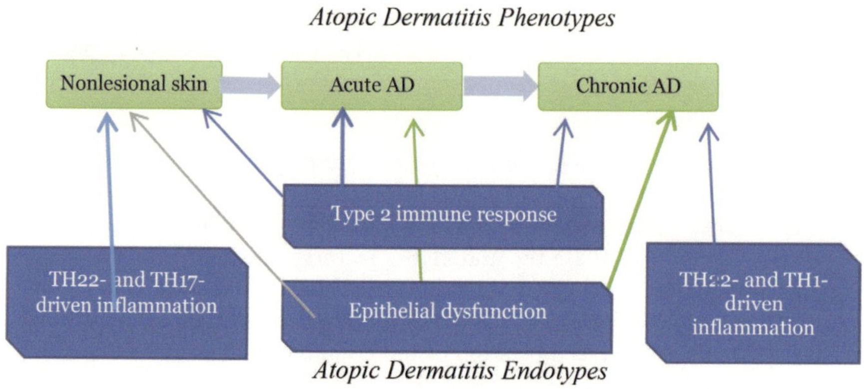

Figure 2.
Proposed atopic dermatitis Endotypes. Adapted from reference [100].

inflammatory processes involving B-cells, T-cells, neutrophils, macrophages and natural killer cells. Inhibitors of this pathway reduce are anti-inflammatory.

5.2 AD clinical phenotypes

AD has variable phenotypes that vary with age of onset, race, clinical course (acute or chronic), disease severity, therapeutic response, reactions to infectious agents, and allergic/irritant substances, IgE reactivity, and presence of other allergic diseases (asthma, allergic rhinitis, and food allergies). [94]

There are three main phenotypes of atopic dermatitis (**Figure 2**): (1) nonlesional skin, (2) acute AD, and (3) chronic remitting relapsing AD with acute flares. The underlying cellular and immune mechanisms in all three phenotypes are based on dysfunctional immune response as well as epithelial disruption. It is believed that underlying these complex clinical phenotypes are biomarkers that can be validated, and qualified for precision medicine for individualized treatment of AD. [100]

(2) non–type 2 immune response AD - with Th1-, Th17-, and Th22-induced inflammatory process and resultant epithelial dysfunction. [101–103]

5.3 Pathological markers

Disease assessment can be done pathologically. Biomarkers, such as CCL17, can be used for assessment of AD severity while filaggrin deficiency is being considered as a potential candidate for prognosticating the disease. Indoleamine 2,3-dioxygenase has been found useful as a predictive marker for viral skin infections [104].

5.4 Triggers for AD onset and exacerbation

Triggers are predisposing factors to AD episodes or flares. The control of these triggers are paramount in the treatment of AD. [105] and in improving the quality of life by maintain a disease free periods for the affected individuals or patients.

Atopic dermatitis may be triggered by microbial agents (common cold, secondary infection of lesions and skin infections), food (commonly due to eggs, milk, peanuts, wheat, soy, tree nuts, and fish and other sea foods), [106] aeroallergens (mostly house dust mites, molds, pollens, cigarette smoke, and animal dander), cosmetics, fragrances, weather (extremes of temperature and sweating), [106, 107] clothing such as wool [108], irritants, and sex hormones. [109] The two types of allergic reactions that can result from these triggers are – (1) Immediate allergic reactions: IgE mediated type III with activation of the complement system, and (2) Delayed allergic reactions: due to activation of T lymphocytes and eosinophils. [110]

A. Microbial agents.

Dysfunctional adaptive immune response resulting in increased total and specific IgE levels, [111, 112] and innate immune system abnormalities such as reduced chemotaxis of cells to skin and antimicrobial peptide levels, Toll-like receptor defects [113] are the underlying factors contributing to skin infection and colonization. Disruption of the epidermal barrier facilitates microbial infection and colonization in AD patients. [114] The skin of AD individuals are highly predisposed to colonization or infection by various organisms most especially *Staphylococcus aureus* and Herpes simplex virus. [115]

The microbial organisms produce superantigens which stimulates marked inflammation. *S. aureus* has been implicated as a trigger of AD and as a factor responsible for chronic relapsing clinical course. [16] It releases toxins and superantigens that stimulates the innate immune response leading to T cells and macrophages production. It has been found in the skin of 80–100% AD individuals. [16] Specific IgE antibodies against staphylococcal enterotoxins corresponding to severity of the disease have been found in most AD cases. [16] The stimulation of chemokines such as TH2 cytokines IL-4 and IL-13 leads to reduced mobilization of human beta-defensin-2 (HBD-2) and impairs keratinocytes clearing of *Staph. aureus* while their neutralization significantly leads to clearance of the infective agent. [115–117] Apart from areas of infection, S aureus also colonizes normal-appearing skin in AD patients. [117]

Viral skin infections occur in AD patients more than other individuals without atopy. These infections may be localized or widespread. The most frequently seen viral infections are herpes simplex, warts and molluscum contagiosum. According to Damour et al., susceptibility is increased by overexpression of Th2 cytokines - IL-4, IL-13, IL-25, IL-33, and TSLP, low the AMP cathelicidin LL-37 and HBD-2 production; reduced IFN-γ, defect in cellular immune response by NK cells and dendritic cells. [115]

HSV may present as umbilicated vesicles, punched out erosions, impetigo-like lesions or secondarily infect atopic skin lesions. [115] Tzanck smear, PCR and viral culture can be used to confirm diagnosis. Also, fungi infection particularly *Malassezia sympodialis* has been found to contribute to chronic inflammation in AD, and it is associated with specific IgE antibodies against *M. sympodialis.* It was found to be more common in patients with head and neck type of AD.

B. Aeroallergens.

Aeroallergens are one of the most common environmental allergens causing AD flares or worsening. Many AD individuals have been found to have delayed hypersensitivity reactions to aeroallergens identified in their environment or reported by the patients while they have no reactions to aeroallergens which they had not been exposed to. Aeroallergens often producing delayed reactions with patch tests in adults AD are house dust mite, pollens (weed, grass and tree), and danders. [118] Adults with IgE sensitization to these aeroallergens have increased risk of developing persistent lesions of AD and other allergic diseases. [119] Control measures such as the use of allergen-impermeable mattress encasing, acaridae spray containing tannic acid and benzylbenzoate has been found to reduce the house dust mite antigen, Der p1. [120]

C. Food allergens.

Food allergy refers to an adverse immune-mediated reaction to ingested food product which is reproducible. [121, 122] Food intolerance is an undesirable non-allergic food reactions that does not involve the immune system (lactose intolerance). Prevalence of FA in adults is about 1–2%. [122] Some double-blind placebo-controlled oral food challenges (DBPCFCs) have shown that FA in adults AD are considerably lesser than in children, may not correlate with skin prick testing (SPT) or patch testing, and there may be little benefit to elimination diets. [123] However, a significant association has been reported between the IgE-mediated food allergy and severity of AD in adults. [124]

The immune reactions are of three types: [122].

a. IgE-mediated (immediate hypersensitivity reaction) - serum specific IgE antibody present with specific symptoms on ingestion of the food allergen within 2 hours. Symptoms include:

   i. Skin symptoms – itching of lips and/or eyes, eye redness, swelling of lips/tongue, urticaria, angioedema, flushing, rash, exacerbation of eczema;

   ii. Gastrointestinal symptoms – nausea, vomiting, diarrhea, pain and bloating;

   iii. Respiratory symptoms – nasal itching, rhinorrhea, sneezing, wheezing, dyspnea, or anaphylaxis;

b. Non-IgE-mediated (T-cell mediated with histological changes); (c) Combined reactions.

The skin is affected in 86% of food allergies and 38% respiratory system involvement. [121] The "priority antigens" which constitutes >90% of FA are dairy products, eggs (chicken), nuts (e.g., hazelnuts, walnuts, almonds, cashews, peanuts), soy beans, fish, crustaceans and shellfish, gluten foods (e.g., wheat, rye, barley), sesame and mustard. [121, 125] Less commonly: legumes, some fruits/juices (e.g., apple, grape), and vegetables (e.g., onions celery, carrots). [125] It is thought that raw food ingestion and food borne microbes may act as antigen. [126] This elicits immune responses by binding to immature gut villus, by increasing gut permeability, and by antigen transfer. [126] Food antigens produce anaphylactic reactions in sensitized individuals due to loss of oral tolerance to these antigens. [127].

Current therapies for FA entails strict avoidance of the offending food and allergen immunotherapy (AIT) - oral immunotherapy (OIT), sublingual immunotherapy (SLIT) and epicutaneous immunotherapy (EPIT) to ensure clinical desensitization, sustained unresponsiveness to allergens, and oral tolerance. [127] SLIT and EPIT are safer and more tolerable than OIT due to lesser ingestion of protein. [128]

6. Clinical features

6.1 Clinical symptoms and signs

Adult AD presentations are variable and differs by age, severity and course of the disease (acute or chronic course). It is a relapsing and remitting condition, with episodes of disease exacerbation that occurs as frequently as two or three times per month. [13] Clinical symptoms and signs of adult/adolescent AD as reported by Liu et al., [129] in a multicenter study (42 dermatological centers) of 1605 AD cases over 12 years old (in decreasing percentages) are:

Pruritus (98.6), Xerosis (74.1), Associated environmental/emotional factors (73.9), Personal or family history of atopic diseases (61.4), Itching upon sweating (56.0), Flexural dermatitis (52.0), Facial pallor/facial erythema (35.5), Intolerance to wool (30.2), Eczema/AD before 12 years old (29.5), Scalp eczema/pityriasis (28.8), Urticaria/angioedema (26.8), Periauricular fissuring/eczema (25.8), Hand and/or foot dermatitis (24.7), Ichthyosis/palmar hyperlinearity/keratosis pilaris (23.3), Eyelid eczema (20.8), Eczema/AD history before 2 years old (20.2), Perifollicular accentuation (19.5), White dermographism (19.0), Nummular eczema (18.4), Pompholyx of hand/foot (17.2), Liable to skin infections (16.8), Anterior neck folds (16.7), Cheilitis (15.0), Perineum eczema (14.3), Orbital darkening (11.4), Pityriasis alba (9.5), Breast eczema (7.9), Recurrent conjunctivitis (7.3), Dennie–Morgan infraorbital fold (6.1), Anterior subcapsular cataracts (3.4), Keratoconus (1.3).

The characteristic sites of distribution of skin symptoms for adult AD are the hands, shoulders, neck, flexures, face and eyelids. The extremities and the trunk were less involved. [11] Adult AD characteristically presents as lichenified eczema on both extensor and flexural surfaces of the flexures, face, neck, shoulders and hands. In elderly adults, eczematous erythroderma is common. [4] Pruritus is a major symptom and major criteria in AD. It increases in the night.

6.2 Clinical patterns of adult AD

Three clinical patterns have been described by Heli et al. [130]

1. Chronic, persistent AD

2. Relapsing course

3. Adult-onset AD

Some classify the clinical features into (a) adult-onset AD, and (b) persistent AD and AD with relapsing course grouped together as persistent/recurring infantile or childhood AD. [131] In the elderly, AD can occur as geriatric onset AD, geriatric recurrence of typical childhood AD, and geriatric recurrence and /or continuation of adult AD. [10]

Persistent AD – refers to childhood AD running a chronic recurrent course up to and even in adulthood; occurs in 20–30% childhood cases. [131] Presentations are similar to children with flexural involvement (flexor surface of extremities) in majority of patients with pre-adult-onset. [132] The flexures are the areas initially involved. The flexor surface of arms and legs are also more highly involved than other body areas in these patients than those with adult-onset adult AD. [132] Affected cases usually have diffuse, lichenified, symmetrical lesions in the flexures mostly with facial eczema, dirty neck, and variable involvement of hands, limbs and trunk. Dirty neck, and vitiligo-like lichenified lesions in the flexures are signs of chronicity. [133–135]

Relapsing AD – this refers to childhood AD with complete resolution before or during adolescence, and recurrence in adulthood; occurs in about 12.2% cases of childhood AD. [131] Adult AD cases are prone to contact hand eczema while few with contact eczema have AD. According to Salvador et al., many of these patients have chronic hand eczema as a result of atopy precipitated by irritant substances (heat, dust, soaps, etc) at work places or jobs causing wet hands. [131] This is often confused with contact irritant dermatitis and it is difficult to distinguish the two. [131, 136–138]

Adult-onset AD – In a study by Son et al., the body-site distribution of areas initially involved showed that the head and neck areas are the sites initially affected at the onset in adult-onset AD in contrast to flexural areas in pre-adult-onset AD. [132] The trunk was the most common area affected while flexural surfaces of arms and legs are the most affected area in persistent AD. [132]

From the study by Tanei et al., the senile-type AD usually have involvement of the face and neck, trunk, lichenification in flexural and extensor surfaces of arms and legs. [139] The antecubital and popliteal surfaces are less affected. Cases with moderate to severe eczema have other features of AD: erythroderma particularly on the face (atopic red face), loss of lateral eyebrows (Hertoghe sign), facial pallor, dirty neck (eczema with reticulate, ripple, or poikilodermic pigmentation), goose skin and Dennie–Morgan infraorbital folds. [139]

Tanei [140], described 3 types of lichenification in the antecubital areas of elderly patients with AD:

a. Localized lichenified eczema in the elbow fold;

b. Diffuse lichenified eczema in the elbow fold and flexure site of the arm;

c. Lichenified eczema around the scarcely involved elbow fold (reverse sign).

In the elderly, the classical type of localized lichenified eczema at elbow and knee folds is less common than the reverse type where lesions are around unaffected folds.

6.3 Clinical assessment of AD in adults

Assessment of AD should be done to determine the appropriate treatment as well as monitor response to therapy. SCORAD – SCORing Atopic Dermatitis – is a clinical tool for assessing the severity (extent/spread, intensity, and symptoms) of atopic dermatitis both objectively and subjectively. [141, 142] It was developed in 1993 by the European Task Force on Atopic Dermatitis to provide a consensus approach to AD management and useful in both children and adults. [143] Intensity of the symptoms was giving a weight of 60% and 20% each was allocated to spread (extent) and subjective signs (insomnia, itch). [144]

It consists of 3 components – A (Area or Extent), B (Intensity), C (Subjective symptoms). The formula for obtaining the total AD score of an individual is $A/5 + 7B/2 + C$. Area is expressed as a percentage of the whole body using the rule of 9 with a maximum value of 100%. Intensity has a maximum of 18 from a score of 6 for each of redness, swelling, oozing/crusting, scratch marks, skin thickening (lichenification), and dryness (assessed in an area where there is no inflammation). Subjective symptoms are itch or sleeplessness assessed on a scale of 0–10 for each with a maximum 20.

7. Diagnostic criteria

Reports of AD in adults are not common and the clinical features are not categorical. However, the diagnosis of atopic dermatitis (AD) is based on its clinical symptoms regardless of age or sex of the individual. According to Tada [8], in the review of AD diagnostic criteria, the first concept of AD was described and published in 1933 by Wise and Sulzberger. [145]

Major criteria (3 or more needed for diagnosis):
1. Pruritus 2. Typical morphology and distribution 3. Flexural lichenification in adults 4. Facial and extensor involvement in infants and children 5. Dermatitis - Chronically or chronically relapsing 6. Personal or family history of atopy (asthma, hay fever, atopic dermatitis)
Minor criteria (3 or more needed for diagnosis):
(1) Xerosis (2) Ichthyosis/palmar hyperlinearity, keratosis pilaris (3) Immediate (type I) skin test reaction (4) Elevated serum IgE (5) Early age of onset (6) Tendency toward cutaneous infections (especially staph. Aureus and herpes simplex), impaired cell mediated immunity (7) Tendency toward non-specific hand or foot dermatitis (8) Nipple eczema (9) Cheilitis (10) Recurrent conjunctivitis (11) Dennie-Morgan infraorbital fold (12) Keratoconus (13) Anterior subcapsular cataracts (14) Orbital darkening (15) Facial pallor, facial erythema (16) Pityriasis alba (17) Anterior neck folds (18) Itch when sweating (19) Intolereance to wool ad lipid solvents (20) Periofollicular accentuation (21) Food intolerance (22) Course influenced by environmental and emotional factors (23) White dermographism, delayed blanch

Table 1.
Hanifin and Rajka diagnostic criteria for atopic dermatitis.

The first diagnostic criteria published was in 1961 by Rajka. [8] Both Hanifin and Rajka modified and combined their criteria in 1980 to form the most commonly used criteria (**Table 1**), [146] and many dermatological societies have also developed their criteria for this condition. According to Tada, the diagnostic standard by Hanifin and Rajka is useful in AD diagnosis in children and it also remains useful in adults as well. It has 6 major and 23 minor criteria.

According to the UK Working Party on AD in childhood, to qualify as a case of atopic dermatitis, the individual must have an itchy skin condition plus three or more of the following: history of flexural involvement, a history of asthma/hay fever, a history of a generalized dry skin, onset of rash under the age of 2 years, or visible flexural dermatitis. This has a sensitivity of 85% and specificity of 96%. [147] AD can consequently be diagnosed mainly by clinical symptoms and signs.

8. Complications

- Impetigo contagiosa
- Eczema herpeticum
- Molluscum contagiosum
- Erythrodermic eczema
- Ocular complication (keratoconus, cataract and/or retinal detachment)
- Kaposi's varicelliform eruption

9. Differential diagnoses

Differentials of adult-onset AD are seborrheic dermatitis, allergic contact dermatitis, cutaneous T-cell lymphoma, polymorphous light eruption, actinic prurigo, and psoriasis, prurigo simplex, scabies, miliaria, ichthyosis, xerotic eczema, hand dermatitis (non-atopic), psoriasis, immunodeficiency diseases, collagen diseases (SLE, dermatomyositis), Netherton syndrome. In children, scabies, tinea corporis, seborrheic dermatitis, nutritional deficiency and allergic contact dermatitis are close differentials. [148]

10. Investigations

Investigations for AD are rarely required. Most investigations are carried out to identify triggering factors where applicable. A skin prick test is used for food and aeroallergen sensitization. Extracts or fresh food, and aeroallergens can be tested by placing them directly on the skin, which is then pricked through the liquid. This can also apply for local foods, which can be crushed with saline and similarly tested. The 'prick-prick test' can also be used by pricking the food with a lancet and then pricking the skin. The test site is observed in 15–20 minutes and the wheal reaction measured and recorded. A positive control with histamine should be ≥3 mm and a negative control is done with normal saline. [149] Patch tests are performed to diagnose allergic contact dermatitis (ACD); or a worsening dermatitis as a result of ACD to a constituent of the topical treatment. [150] Patch test is done for superimposed allergic contact dermatitis; in cases of suspected hand dermatitis. The highly specific atopy patch test is used to diagnose type IV hypersensitivity reactions.

Skin biopsy is usually required when there is erythroderma and a need to identify the underlying etiology. Histological findings can be suggestive of AD; however, they are not reliable for making a diagnosis. Total serum IgE levels are not specific for AD and does not correlate with disease severity. It is elevated in 50% of cases of AD.

In adult AD, colonization with *Staphylococcus aureus* is high and adult skin is more heavily colonized with Malassezia yeasts. [4] A positive ImmunoCAP assay for Malassezia species may be carried out. [149] This can then be treated with appropriate oral therapy. Swab tests can be carried out where necessary for secondary bacterial infections. Other tests are carried out appropriately based on other associated findings from the history or clinical examination.

11. Management

A very important part of management of AD is the education and counseling of all AD patients. With good understanding of the disease and what aggravates it, disease control can be achieved with the right skin care plan and an understanding of how to manage the flares. Successful management requires identification, elimination and prevention of specific identifiable and non-identifiable trigger factors. Managing AD requires a multispecialty approach which involves the dermatologist, allergologist, psychologist and nutritionist. Treatment regimens are usually based on the severity of the condition (**Table 2**). Evaluation and treatment according to ETFAD/EADV Eczema task force 2020 consensus paper is useful in routine clinical practice for AD in adults. [7] Patients should be educated on all available therapeutic options and they must actively participate in choosing the best option for themselves and their circumstance. Treatment regimens should be discussed and explained to individuals and their families to ensure adherence and compliance. Expectations, limitations, therapeutic options and prognosis are key to the overall management of AD.

Topical treatment.

The use of emollients is required both during an acute phase and as maintenance therapy as it forms the cornerstone of treatment for all types and severity of AD.

General measures	Mild	Moderate	Severe
Educate patients	Mildly potent TCS	Moderately potent TCS	Potent TCS
Emollients	TCIs	Crisaborole	Short course: OCS
Bath oils	Crisaborole	Wet wrap therapy	Short course: Cyclosporine A
Avoid triggers		NB-UVB/PUVA1	Biologics: Dupilumab
Antihistamines (Sedating type)			Long course: azathioprine, MMF
Antibiotics			Phototherapy: PUVA1
Bandages			

Table 2.
The treatment recommendations according to severity in adult AD.

Therapeutic baths in salt-rich water, colloidal oatmeal, wet –wrap dressings and topical antibiotics play an important role in this part of AD treatment.

Topical corticosteroids (TCS) are mainly used during a flare (**Table 3**). There are various potencies and dosages which are used based on severity of AD. TCS are used in active disease for up to 4 weeks and then 2 to 3 times weekly for preventive treatment. Topical calcineurin inhibitors (TCIs) are recommended for maintenance. Tacrolimus is more effective than pimecrolimus, and has been shown to be effective and well tolerated. [150–152] TCIs suppresses calcineurin which stimulates the expression of interleukin 2 (IL-2), a cytokine that regulates the T cell response. TCIs inhibit mast cell and neutrophil activation, basophil, eosinophil, and Langerhans cells functions.

Crisaborole, a topical phosphodiesterase-4 (PDE-4) inhibitor which downregulates the T-cell signaling pathways by inhibiting cAMP degradation is effective in reducing skin inflammation. [153]

Other forms of topical therapy include therapeutic baths in salt-rich water or colloidal oatmeal; diluted bleach baths and wet –wrap dressings and topical antibiotic when required.

Phototherapy can be used for moderate to severe AD, particularly where topical therapy has failed. Narrow band UVB in combination with medium dose UVA is

Severity	Eruption	TCS application
Severe	Primarily severe swelling/ edema /infiltration or erythema with lichenification, multiple papules, severe scales, crusts, vesicles, erosion, multiple excoriations and pruriginous nodules	Use of very strong or strong rank TCS is the first-line treatment. Strongest rank TCS are also available for refractory pruriginous nodules if sufficient effects are not achieved by applying very strong rank TCS
Moderate	Primarily moderate erythema, scales, a few papules and excoriations	Use of strong or medium rank TCS is the first-line treatment
Mild	Primarily dryness, mild erythema and scales	Use of strong or medium rank TCS is the first-line treatment
Slight	Primarily dryness with negligible inflammation	Topical application of medicines other than TCS (emollients)

Table 3.
Severity of eruption and topical corticosteroid (TCS) application. TCS, topical corticosteroid. [cited from Japanese guidelines for atopic dermatitis 2020. https://doi.org/10.1016/j.alit.2020.02.006, an open access article under the terms of the http://creativecommons.org/licenses/by-nc-nd/4.0/].

effective. [154–156] This mode of treatment however does have long term adverse effects (skin malignancies), and may not be available in all settings.

Systemic treatment (Dosages and side effects cited from Megna et al.) [157].

AD is being recognized as a systemic disease with atopic and nonatopic comorbidities. This plays an important role in the subsequent management and therapeutic implications for this condition.

Systemic therapy is required for chronic, severe cases, resistant cases, and when topical therapy has failed to control the disease. These include antihistamines, oral corticosteroids, immunosuppressive drugs and biologics. Combination of both topical and systemic is indicated for severe and resistant cases. [157]

Antihistamines may help to reduce itching. [158] Hydroxyzine and diphenhydramine hydrochloride provide a certain degree of relief but are not effective without other treatments.

Erythromycin, clarithromycin or cephalosporins can be used for 7–10 days for widespread bacterial skin infections. They are not recommended for use where there is no evidence of clinical infection as staphylococcal organisms are known to colonize the skin of AD patients. Systemic antifungals - itraconazole and ketoconazole – useful for cases with *Malassezia sympodialis* infection. [159]

1. Non-biologic drugs (Immunosuppressant and other)

    a. Oral corticosteroids (OCS) are effective for short term treatment for acute flares (**Table 2**) OCS rapidly improve the clinical symptoms of AD and are best used for short courses up to 1 week. [157] Long term use of oral steroids is not recommended because of the well-known side effects associated with them. These include hypertension, gastric ulcers, osteoporosis, diabetes and Cushing syndrome; as well as a rebound flare which can occur when they are abruptly stopped. They should be tapered to avoid relapse and rebound of AD. [157, 159–161] Dosage: Varies with type, AD severity, and comorbidities). Important Side effects: Diabetes, hypertension, skin atrophy, gastric ulcer, osteoporosis, glaucoma, pigmentary changes on prolonged use, and Cushing syndrome.

    b. Cyclosporine is the most widely used and first choice of systemic agents for the control of AD not responding to topical therapy. It is an immunomodulatory drug that inhibits interleukin by selective inhibition of cytokine transcription in activated T lymphocyte. Those on cyclosporine require close monitoring to avoid common side effects (nephrotoxicity, tremors, hypertension, electrolyte imbalances, etc.). Baseline tests and regular monitoring is required; particularly their renal status. Cyclosporine remains the only approved drug for systemic treatment of adult AD. Dosage: 2.5 to 5 mg/kg/day. Important Side effects: Nephrotoxicity, Hypertension, nausea, diarrhea, headache, paresthesia and myalgias.

    c. Methotrexate is effective in the treatment for moderate to severe AD. AD control be achieved with at a low dose for prolonged periods without any significant risk to the patient. It is a relatively safe drug. [162] Dosage: 5–25 mg/week. Important Side effects: Liver dysfunction, gastrointestinal complaints, hematological abnormalities, fatigue, and headache.

    d. Azathioprine is a purine synthesis inhibitor that reduces leukocyte proliferation. Various studies have been carried out with varying results.

It is used off label in situations where cyclosporine is contraindicated, or there has been no response. Dosage: 2–3 mg/kg twice a day. Important Side effects: Gastrointestinal disturbances, liver dysfunction, and leucopenia.

e. Others:

i. Mycophenolic mofetil (MMF) - Dosage: MMF:1000–2000 mg/day; EC-MPA enteric-coated mychophenolate sodium: 1440 mg/day. Side effects: Gastrointestinal disturbances, liver dysfunction, fatigue, hematological abnormalities and flu-like syndrome.

ii. Alitretinoin - Dosage: 30 mg/day. Side effects: Headache, TSH elevation, teratogenicity

2. Biologics

This class of pharmacological agents are engineered to target specific mediators of inflammation. Over the past decade, studies have reported the efficacy of targeted therapy blocking cytokines or mediators which play a role in AD pathogenesis. [163] According to Deleanu et al., based on mechanism of action, novel biologic therapies are classified into: anti IL-4 (Dupilumab) and anti-IL-4/IL-13 agents (Lebrikizumab, Tralokinumab), IgE directed therapy (Omalizumab), IL-22 blockers (Fezakinumab), anti-IL-12/23 (Ustekinumab), IL-31 directed therapy (Nemolizumab), thymic stromal lymphopoietin directed therapy (Tezepelumab), phosphodiesterase inhibitors (Apremilast, Crisaborole), and JAK inhibitors (Tofacitinib). [163]

a. Rituximab (anti-CD20) is a monoclonal antibody against the protein CD20, which is primarily found on the surface of immune system B cells. [157] It reduces the expression of IL-5 and IL-13 by lowering B cell activation of T-cells. [164] Data on its use in adult patients with severe AD is limited. [157, 165] Dosage: 500–1000 mg iv (2-cycle infusion 2 weeks apart). Side effects: Headache, fever, nausea, diarrhea, weakness, flushing, muscle or joint pain, increased risk of infection, hematological abnormalities

b. Dupilumab, (anti-CD20) is a human monoclonal antibody that targets the shared α subunit of the IL-4 and IL-13 receptors, effectively blocking Th2 immune response. It is the only biologic drug licensed for treatment of adult AD. Clinical trials (Phase I-III) demonstrated its efficacy, as well as good patient and clinical reported outcomes using the SCORAD, IGA, DLQI and EASI assessment tools and health related quality of life (HRQoL) measures. [166] Long term use and safety profile still need to be established from ongoing studies. Dosage: 300 mg every 1–2 weeks. Side effects: Increased risk of infection, headache, and gastrointestinal disturbances.

c. Others:

i. Interferon-γ and infliximab have been used in severe AD and there are limited studies on their use. [163–165]

ii. Ustekinumab (anti IL-12, IL-23) 45 mg for patients ≤100 kg; 90 mg for patients >100 kg; at weeks 0 and 4 then every

12 weeks. Side effects: Headache, myalgia, increased risk of infection, fatigue, injection site reactions.

iii. Omalizumab (anti-IgE): Dosage: 150–600 mg every 2–4 weeks Side effects: Increased risk of infection, injection site reactions, headache

3. Small molecules

Apremilast is a new drug involved in modulation of multiple anti-inflammatory pathways targeting phosphodiesterase type IV (PDE4) inhibition. Apremilast downregulates pro-inflammatory transcription of several cytokines such as TNF-α, IFN-γ, IL-2, IL-5, IL-8 and IL-12. [163] There are limited studies and data on its use in AD. Dosage: 20–30 mg twice a day. Side effects: Headache, nausea, diarrhea.

Ultraviolet (UV) therapy [157] has the following functions:

- reduces the number of epidermal nerve fibers and expression of axon guidance molecules reducing itching,
- upregulates production of FoxP3-positive regulatory T cells thereby reducing AD severity
- inhibit DNA synthesis hence keratinocyte proliferation,
- suppresses antigen-presenting cells such as Langerhans' cells,
- induces T lymphocyte apoptosis and
- suppresses anti-inflammatory mediator production

It is often used as second-line treatment for moderate-to-severe AD, resistant/relapse, chronic and poor topical response cases.

Broadband useful in adult AD: UVB (290–320 nm), narrow-band (NB) UVB (311–313 nm), excimer laser (308 nm), UVA-1 (340–400 nm), psoralens and UVA (PUVA), and combined UVA/UVB (280–400 nm).Narrow-band UVB radiation and medium-dose UVA1 are the most effective and safe for short and long term treatment.. Medium-dose UVA1 is the only type used in acute flares. Therapy is usually thrice weekly. Known side effects are nausea, fatigue, headache, itching, skin burns, blistering, erythema, irregular pigmentation, photodamage, actinic keratosis, and herpes virus reactivation as well as a higher risk of skin cancer, premature photoaging and skin cancers.

12. Conclusion

There is a worldwide increase in Adult AD with no standardized guidelines for its management. This condition greatly affects the quality of life of individuals and side effects from some of the drugs further limit the long term use of some forms of treatment. Biologic therapies are likely to change the course of the disease: decrease exacerbations, increase flare free periods and improve the quality of life. International guidelines therefore need to be developed based on further research on systemic immunotherapy options.

13. Pictures

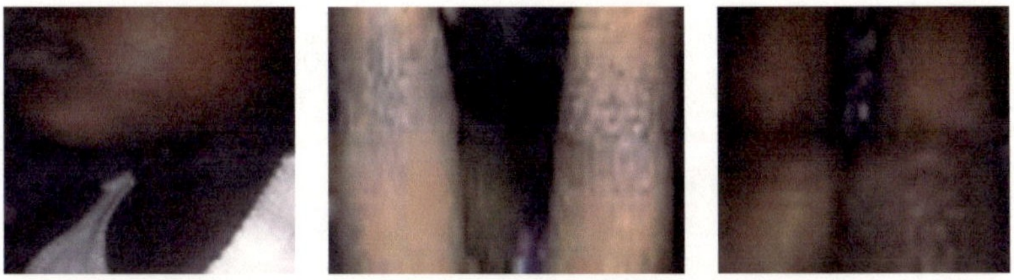

Atopic Dermatitis in a male child with flexural involvement.

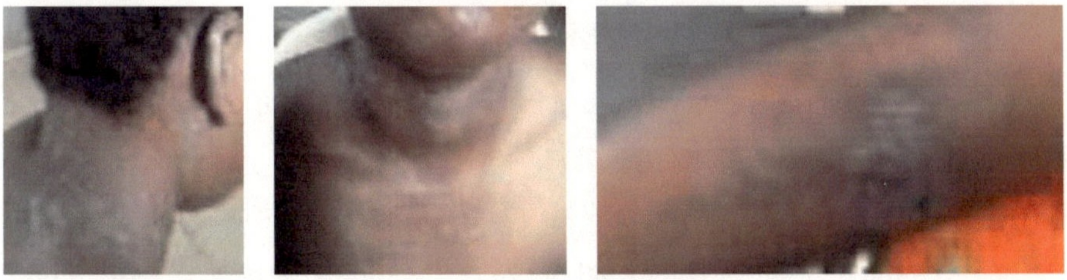

Atopic Dermatitis in a young adult female with involvement of head, neck, and extensor surfaces of elbows.

Author details

Olumayowa Abimbola Oninla[1*], Ayesha Omolara Akinkugbe[2], Bolaji Ibiesa Otike-Odibi[3], Mufutau Muphy Oripelaye[1] and Fatai Olatunde Olanrewaju[1]

1 Department of Dermatology and Venereology, Faculty of Clinical Sciences, College of Health Sciences, Obafemi Awolowo University, Ile-Ife, Osun State, Nigeria

2 Department of Medicine, Dermatology and Genitourinary Medicine Unit, College of Medicine, University of Lagos, Lagos State, Nigeria

3 Department of Internal Medicine, Dermatology Unit, University of Port-Harcourt, Rivers State, Nigeria

*Address all correspondence to: mayooni@yahoo.com

References

[1] Hunter J, Savin, J, Dahl M, eds. Clinical Dermatology. 3rd ed. Massachusetts, USA: Blackwell Science Ltd; 2002.

[2] Kanwar AJ. Adult-onset Atopic Dermatitis. Indian J Dermatol 2016 Nov-Dec;61(6):662–663. doi: 10.4103/0019-5154.193679. PMID: 27904186; PMCID: PMC5122283.

[3] Bannister MJ, Freeman S. Adult-onset atopic dermatitis. Australas J Dermatol 2000;41:225–8.

[4] Katsarou A, Armenaka M. Atopic dermatitis in older patients: particular points. J Eur Acad Dermatol Venereol 2010;25(1):12–8. doi:10.1111/j.1468-3083.2010.03737.x.

[5] Atopy Definition. American Academy of Allergy Asthma & Immunology. [Cited November 7, 2020] Available at: https://www.aaaai.org/conditions-and-treatments/conditions-dictionary/atopy#:~:text=Atopy%20refers%20to%20the%20genetic,inhaled%20allergens%20and%20food%20allergens.

[6] Ring J, Przybilla B, Ruzicka T. Handbook of Atopic Eczema, 2nd edn. Springer, Berlin, 2005.

[7] Wollenberg A, Barbarot S, Bieber T, et al. Consensus-based European guidelines for treatment of atopic eczema (atopic dermatitis) in adults and children: part II. J Eur Acad Dermatol Venereol 2018;32(6):850–878. doi: 10.1111/jdv.14888.

[8] Tada J. Diagnostic Standard for Atopic Dermatitis JMAJ. 2002;45(11): 460–5.

[9] Thomsen SF, Ulrik CS, Kyvik KO. Importance of genetic factors in the etiology of atopic dermatitis: A twin study. Allergy & Asthma Proceedings. 2007;28(5):535–539.

[10] Tanei R, Hasegawa Y, Sawabe M. Abundant immunoglobulin E-positive cells in skin lesions support an allergic etiology of atopic dermatitis in the elderly. J Eur Acad Dermatol Venereol. 2013;27:952–960. DOI: 10.1111/j.1468-3083.2012.04612.x

[11] Pónyai G, Hidvégi B, Németh I, Sas A, Temesvári E, Kárpáti S. Contact and aeroallergens in adulthood atopic dermatitis. J Eur Acad Dermatol Venereol. 2008;22(11):1346–1355. doi: 10.1111/j.1468-3083.2008.02886.x.

[12] Kim J, Lee S, Woo SY, et al. The indoor level of house dust mite allergen is associated with severity of atopic dermatitis in children. J Korean Med Sci. 2013;28(1):74–79. doi:10.3346/jkms.2013.28.1.74.

[13] Sharma A, Loffeld A. The management of eczema in children. Paediatr Child Health. 2014(Sept.);25(2):54–59. DOI:https://doi.org/10.1016/j.paed.2014.08.002

[14] Oninla OA, Oninla SO, Olasode OA, Onayemi O. Pattern of paediatric dermatoses at Dermatology clinics in Ile-Ife and Ilesha, Nigeria. PIntCH. 2016 Jan 29. Available from http://dx.doi.org/10.1080/20469047.2015.1109243.

[15] Ayanlowo O, Puddicombe O, Gold-Olufadi S. Pattern of skin diseases amongst children attending a dermatology clinic in Lagos, Nigeria. Pan Afr Med J. 2018;29:162. doi: 10.11604/pamj.2018.29.162.14503. Available online at: https://www.panafrican-med-journal.com/content/article/29/162/full.

[16] Orfali RL, Shimizu MM, Takaoka R, Zaniboni MC, Ishizaki AS, Costa AA. et al. Atopic dermatitis in adults: clinical and epidemiological considerations. Rev. Assoc. Med. Bras. [Internet]. 2013 June [cited 2020 July 24]; 59(3):270–275.

[17] Silverberg J. Adult-onset Atopic Dermatitis. J Allergy Clin Immunol. Pract. 2019;7(1):28–33. https://doi.org/10.1016/j.jaip.2018.09.029.

[18] Bannister MJ, Freeman S. Adult-onset atopic dermatitis. Australas J Dermatol. 2000;41(4):225–228. doi: 10.1046/j.1440-0960.2000.00442.x.

[19] Mortz CG, Andersen KE, Dellgren C, Barington T, Bindslev-Jensen C. Atopic dermatitis from adolescence to adulthood in the TOACS cohort: prevalence, persistence and comorbidities. Allergy. 2015 Jul;70(7): 836–845. DOI: 10.1111/all.12619.

[20] Leung DYM. Pathogenesis of atopic dermatitis. J Allergy Clin Immunol. 1999;104:3(S99-S108). DOI:https://doi.org/10.1016/S0091-6749(99)70051-5.

[21] Engman MF, Weiss RS, Engman ME Jr. Eczema and environment. Med Clin North Am. 1936;20:651–663.

[22] Nassif A, Chan S, Storrs F, Hanifin J. Abnormal skin irritancy in atopic dermatitis and in atopy without dermatitis. Arch Dermatol 1994;130: 1402–1407.

[23] Saurat J-H. Eczema in primary immune-deficiencies: clues to the pathogenesis of atopic dermatitis with special reference to the Wiskott-Aldrich syndrome. Acta Derm Venereol. 1985; 114:125–128.

[24] Sehra S, Tuana FMB, Holbreich M, Mousdicas N, Kaplan MH, Travers JB. Clinical correlations of recent developments in the pathogenesis of atopic dermatitis. An Bras Dermatol. [Internet]. 2008;83(1): 57–73. Available from: http://www.scielo.br/scielo.php?script=sci_arttext&pid=S0365-05962008000100009&lng=en. http://dx.doi.org/10.1590/S0365-05962008000100009.

[25] Brunner PM, Leung DY, Guttman-Yassky E. Immunologic, microbial, and epithelial interactions in atopic dermatitis. Ann Allergy Asthma Immunol. 2018;120:34–41.

[26] Kim HJ, Baek J, Lee JR, Roh JY, Jung Y. Optimization of cytokine milieu to reproduce atopic dermatitis-related gene expression in HaCaT keratinocyte cell line. Immune Netw 2018;18:e9.

[27] Sullivan M, Silverberg NB. Current and emerging concepts in atopic dermatitis pathogenesis. Clin Dermatol 2017;35(4):349–353. doi:10.1016/j.clindermatol.2017.03.006.

[28] Johansson C, Tengvall LM, Aalberse RC, Scheynius A. Elevated levels of IgG and IgG4 to Malassezia allergens in atopic eczema patients with IgE reactivity to Malassezia. Int Arch Allergy Immunol. 2004;135:93–100.

[29] Schafer T, Heinrich J, Wjst M, Adam H, Ring J, Wichmann HE. Association between severity of atopic eczema and degree of sensitization to aeroallergens in schoolchildren. J Allergy Clin Immunol. 1999;104:1280–4.

[30] Olesen AB, Ellingsen AR, Olesen H, Juul S, Thestrup-Pedersen K. Atopic dermatitis and birth factors: historical follow up by record linkage. BMJ. 1997; 314:1003–8.

[31] Williams HC. Atopic dermatitis: new information from epidemiological studies. Br J Hosp Med. 1994;52:409–12.

[32] Kusel MM, Holt PG, de Klerk N, Sly PD. Support for 2 variants of eczema. J Allergy Clin Immunol. 2005; 116:1067–72.

[33] Sabat R, Wolk K, Loyal L, Döcke W, Ghoreschi K. T cell pathology in skin inflammation. Semin Immunopathol 41, 359–377 (2019). https://doi.org/10.1007/s00281-019-00742-7.

[34] Uehara M, Kimura C (1993) Descendant family history of atopic

dermatitis. Acta Derm Venereol 73: 62–63.

[35] Kypriotou M, Huber M, Hohl D. "The human epidermal differentiation complex: cornified envelope precursors, S100 proteins and the 'fused genes' family". Experimental Dermatology. 2012;21(9):643–9. doi:10.1111/j.1600-0625.2012.01472.x. PMID 22507538. S2CID 5435031.

[36] Marshall D, Hardman MJ, Nield KM, Byrne C. Differentially expressed late constituents of the epidermal cornified envelope. Proc Natl Acad Sci U S A. 2001;98:13031–6.

[37] Mischke D, Korge BP, Marenholz I, Volz A, Ziegler A. Genes encoding structural proteins of epidermal cornification and S100 calcium-binding proteins form a gene complex ("epidermal differentiation complex") on human chromosome 1q21. J Invest Dermatol. 1996;106:989–92.

[38] Palmer CN, Irvine AD, Terron-Kwiatkowski A, Zhao Y, Liao H, Lee SP, et al. Common loss-of-function variants of the epidermal barrier protein filaggrin are a major predisposing factor for atopic dermatitis. Nat Genet. 2006; 38:441–6.

[39] Markova NG, Marekov LN, Chipev CC, Gan SQ, Idler WW, Steinert PM (January 1993). "Profilaggrin is a major epidermal calcium-binding protein". Molecular and Cellular Biology. 13 (1): 613–25. doi:10.1128/MCB.13.1.613. PMC 358940. PMID 8417356.

[40] Candi E, Schmidt R, Melino G. The cornified envelope: a model of cell death in the skin. Nat Rev Mol Cell Biol. 2005; 6:328–40.

[41] Smith FJ, Irvine AD, Terron-Kwiatkowski A, Sandilands A, Campbell LE, Zhao Y, et al. Loss-of-function mutations in the gene encoding filaggrin cause ichthyosis vulgaris. Nat Genet. 2006;38:337–42.

[42] Addor FA, Takaoka R, Rivitti EA, Aoki V (2012) Atopic dermatitis: correlation between non-damaged skin barrier function and disease activity. Int J Dermatol 51:672–676.

[43] Pellerin L, Henry J, Hsu CY, et al. Defects of filaggrin-like proteins in both lesional and nonlesional atopic skin. J Allergy Clin Immunol 2013;131(4): 1094–1102. doi:10.1016/j.jaci.2012.12.1566.

[44] Kusari A, Han AM, Schairer D, Eichenfield LF. Atopic dermatitis: New developments. Dermatol Clin 2019;37: 11–20.

[45] Bao L, Mohan GC, Alexander JB, et al. A molecular mechanism for IL-4 suppression of loricrin transcription in epidermal keratinocytes: Implication for atopic dermatitis pathogenesis. Innate Immun 2017;23:641–647.

[46] Nguyen M, Pona A, Kolli SS, Feldman SR, Strowd LC. Recent insights in atopic dermatitis pathogenesis, treatment, and disease impact. J Dermatol Dermatol Surg 2019;23:66–72.

[47] Danso M, Boiten W, van Drongelen V, et al. Altered expression of epidermal lipid bio-synthesis enzymes in atopic dermatitis skin is accompanied by changes in stratum corneum lipid composition. J Dermatol Sci 2017;88: 57–66.

[48] Danso MO, van Drongelen V, Mulder A, et al. TNF-α and Th2 cytokines induce atopic dermatitis-like features on epidermal differentiation proteins and stratum corneum lipids in human skin equivalents. J Invest Dermatol 2014; 134:1941–1950.

[49] Berdyshev E, Goleva E, Bronova I, et al. Lipid abnormalities in atopic skin are driven by type 2 cytokines. JCI Insight

2018;3(4):e98006. Published 2018 Feb 22. doi:10.1172/jci.insight.98006.

[50] Lowe AJ, Leung DYM, Tang MLK, Su JC, and Allen KJ. The skin as a target for prevention of the atopic march. Ann Allergy Asthma Immunol. 2018; 120: 145–151.

[51] Egawa G, and Kabashima K. Multifactorial skin barrier deficiency and atopic dermatitis: Essential topics to prevent the atopic march. J Allergy Clin Immunol. 2016; 138:350–358.e1.

[52] Schleimer RP, and Berdnikovs S. Etiology of epithelial barrier dysfunction in patients with type 2 inflammatory diseases. J Allergy Clin Immunol 2017; 139:1752–1761.

[53] Günzel D, Yu AS. Claudins and the modulation of tight junction permeability. Physiol Rev 2013;93(2): 525–569. doi:10.1152/physrev. 00019.2012

[54] Kaufman BP, Guttman-Yassky E, and Alexis AF. Atopic dermatitis in diverse racial and ethnic groups-Variations in epidemiology, genetics, clinical presentation and treatment. Exp Dermatol 2018; 27:340–357.

[55] Irvine AD, McLean WH, and Leung DY. Filaggrin mutations associated with skin and allergic diseases. N Engl J Med 2011;365:1315–1327.

[56] Bin L, and Leung DY. Genetic and epigenetic studies of atopic dermatitis. Allergy Asthma Clin Immunol 2016; 12:52.

[57] Namkung JH, Lee JE, Kim E, et al. Association of polymorphisms in genes encoding IL-4. IL-13 and their receptors with atopic dermatitis in a Korean population. Exp Dermatol 2011;20: 915–919.

[58] Esaki H, Ewald DA, Ungar B, et al. Identification of novel immune and barrier genes in atopic dermatitis by means of laser capture microdissection. J Allergy Clin Immunol 2015;135:153–163.

[59] Lee YL, Yen JJ, Hsu LC, et al. Association of STAT6 genetic variants with childhood atopic dermatitis in Taiwanese population. J Dermatol Sci 2015; 79:222–228.

[60] Salpietro C, Rigoli L, Miraglia Del Giudice M, et al. TLR2 and TLR4 gene polymorphisms and atopic dermatitis in Italian children: a multicenter study. Int J Immunopathol Pharmacol 2011; 24 (Suppl):33–40.

[61] Suzuki H, Makino Y, Nagata M, et al. A rare variant in CYP27A1 and its association with atopic dermatitis with high serum total IgE. Allergy. 2016; 71: 1486–1489.

[62] Heine G, Hoefer N, Franke A, et al. Association of vitamin D receptor gene polymorphisms with severe atopic dermatitis in adults. Br J Dermatol. 2013; 168:855–858.

[63] Salimi M, Barlow JL, Saunders SP, et al. A role for IL-25 and IL-33–driven type-2 innate lymphoid cells in atopic dermatitis. Exp Med 2013;210:2939–2950. https://doi.org/10.1084/jem. 20130351

[64] Gittler JK, Shemer A, Suárez-Fariñas M, et al. Progressive activation of T(H)2/T(H)22 cytokines and selective epidermal proteins characterizes acute and chronic atopic dermatitis. J Allergy Clin Immunol. 2012;130(6):1344–1354. doi:10.1016/j.jaci.2012.07.012.

[65] Beck LA, Thaçi D, Hamilton JD, Graham LM, Bieber T, Rocklin R, et. al. Dupilumab Treatment in Adults with Moderate-to-Severe Atopic Dermatitis. N Engl J Med 2014; 371:130–139. DOI: 10.1056/NEJMoa1314768.

[66] Brandt EB, Sivaprasad U. Th2 cytokines and atopic dermatitis. J Clin Cell Immunol 2011;2. pii: 110.

[67] Gadani S, Cronk JC, Norris GT, Kipnis J. Interleukin-4: A Cytokine to Remember. J Immunol 2012;189(9):4213–19. DOI:10.4049/jimmunol.1202246. PMC 3481177. PMID 23087426.

[68] Nguyen M, Pona A, Kolli SS, Feldman SR, Strowd LC. Recent insights in atopic dermatitis pathogenesis, treatment, and disease impact. J Dermatol Dermatol Surg 2019;23:66–72.

[69] Nowicka D, Grywalska E. The role of immune defects and colonization of *Staphylococcus aureus* in the pathogenesis of atopic dermatitis. Anal Cell Pathol (Amst) 2018;2018:1956403.

[70] Guttman-Yassky E, Krueger JG, Lebwohl MG. Systemic immune mechanisms in atopic dermatitis and psoriasis with implications for treatment. Exp Dermatol 2018;27:409–17.

[71] Sehra S, Yao Y, Howell MD, et al. IL-4 regulates skin homeostasis and the predisposition toward allergic skin inflammation. J Immunol 2010;184(6): 3186–3190. doi:10.4049/jimmunol.0901860.

[72] Hönzke S, Wallmeyer L, Ostrowski A, Radbruch M, Mundhenk L, Schäfer-Korting M, et al. Influence of Th2 cytokines on the cornified envelope, tight junction proteins, and ß-defensins in filaggrin-deficient skin equivalents. J Invest Dermatol 2016;136:631–9.

[73] Izuhara K, Nunomura S, Nanri Y, Ogawa M, Ono J, Mitamura Y, et al. Periostin in inflammation and allergy. Cell Mol Life Sci 2017;74:4293–303.

[74] Boguniewicz M. Biologic therapy for atopic dermatitis: moving beyond the practice parameter and guidelines. J Allergy Clin Immunol Pract 2017; 5: 1477–1487.

[75] Howell MD, Kim BE, Gao P, et al. Cytokine modulation of atopic dermatitis filaggrin skin expression. J Allergy Clin Immunol 2009; 124: R7–R12.

[76] Gavrilova T. Immune dysregulation in the pathogenesis of atopic dermatitis. Dermatitis 2018;29:57–62.

[77] Perrigoue JG, Zaph C, Guild K, Du Y, Artis D. IL-31-IL-31R interactions limit the magnitude of Th2 cytokine-dependent immunity and inflammation following intestinal helminth infection. J Immunol. 2009;182(10):6088–6094. doi:10.4049/jimmunol.0802459.

[78] Furue M, Yamamura K, Kido-Nakahara M, Nakahara T, Fukui Y. Emerging role of interleukin-31 and interleukin-31 receptor in pruritusin atopic dermatitis. Allergy 2018;73: 29–36.

[79] Leonardi S, Cuppari C, Manti S, et al. Serum interleukin 17,interleukin 23, and interleukin 10 values in children with atopic eczema/dermatitis syndrome (AEDS): association with clinical severity and phenotype. Allergy Asthma Proc. 2015;36:74–81.

[80] Rebane A, Zimmermann M, Aab A, Baurecht H, Koreck A, Karelson M, et al. Mechanisms of IFN-gamma-induced apoptosis of human skin keratinocytes in patients with atopic dermatitis. J Allergy Clin Immunol 2012;129:1297–306.

[81] Sgnotto FD, de Oliveira MG, Lira AA, Inoue AH, Titz TO, Orfali RL, et al. IgG from atopic dermatitis patients induces IL-17 and IL-10 production in infant intrathymic TCD4 and TCD8 cells. Int J Dermatol 2018;57:434–40.

[82] Hennino A, Jean-Decoster C, Giordano-Labadie F, Debeer S, Vanbervliet B, Rozieres A, et al. CD81 T cells are recruited early to allergen exposure sites in atopy patch test reactions in human atopic dermatitis. J Allergy Clin Immunol 2011;127:10647.

[83] Castro F, Cardoso AP, Gonçalves RM, Serre K, Oliveira MJ. Interferon-Gamma at the Crossroads of Tumor Immune Surveillance or Evasion. Front. Immunol. 2018;9:847 DOI= 10.3389/fimmu.2018.00847.

[84] Werfel T, Morita A, Grewe M, et al. Allergen specificity of skin-infiltrating T cells is not restricted to a type-2 cytokine pattern in chronic skin lesions of atopic dermatitis. J Invest Dermatol. 1996;107(6):871–876. doi:10.1111/1523-1747.ep12331164.

[85] Czarnowicki T, Esaki H, Gonzalez J, et al. Early pediatric atopic dermatitis shows only a cutaneous lymphocyte antigen (CLA)(+) TH2/TH1 cell imbalance, whereas adults acquire CLA (+) TH22/TC22 cell subsets. J Allergy Clin Immunol 2015;136(4):941–951.e3. doi:10.1016/j.jaci.2015.05.049.

[86] Werfel T. The role of leukocytes, keratinocytes, and allergen-specific IgE in the development of atopic dermatitis. J Invest Dermatol 2009;129:1878–91.

[87] Hijnen D, Knol EF, Gent YY, Giovannone B, Beijn SJ, Kupper TS, et al. CD8(1) T cells in the lesional skin of atopic dermatitis and psoriasis patients are an important source of IFN-gamma, IL-13, IL-17, and IL-22. J Invest Dermatol 2013;133:973–9.

[88] Hennino A, Jean-Decoster C, Giordano-Labadie F, Debeer S, Vanbervliet B, Rozieres A, et al. CD81 T cells are recruited early to allergen exposure sites in atopy patch test reactions in human atopic dermatitis. J Allergy Clin Immunol 2011;127:1064–7.

[89] Czarnowicki T, Gonzalez J, Shemer A, Malajian D, Xu H, Zheng X, et al. Severe atopic dermatitis is characterized by selective expansion of circulating TH2/TC2 and TH22/TC22, but not TH17/TC17, cells within the skin-homing T-cell population. J Allergy Clin Immunol 2015;136:104–15.e7.

[90] Sua'rez-Farin˜as M, Dhingra N, Gittler J, et al. Intrinsic atopic dermatitis shows similar TH2 and higher TH17 immune activationcompared with extrinsic atopic dermatitis. J Allergy Clin Immunol. 2013; 132:361–370.

[91] Tan Q, Yang H, Liu E, and Wang H. P38/ERK MAPK signaling pathways are involved in the regulation of filaggrin and involucrin by IL-17. Mol Med Rep. 2017; 16:8863–8867.

[92] Eyerich K, Pennino D, Scarponi C, et al. IL-17 in atopic eczema: linking allergen-specific adaptive and microbial-triggered innate immune response. J Allergy Clin Immunol. 2009; 123(1):59–66.e4. doi:10.1016/j.jaci.2008.10.031

[93] O'Regan GM, Sandilands A, McLean WHI, Irvine AD. Filaggrin in atopic dermatitis. J. Allergy Clin. Immunol 2009;124:S2, R2-R6. doi:https://doi.org/10.1016/j.jaci.2009.07.013.

[94] Wambre E, DeLong JH, James EA, LaFond RE, Robinson D, Kwok WW. Differentiation stage determines pathologic and protective allergen-specific CD41 Tcell outcomes during specific immunotherapy. J Allergy Clin Immunol 2012;129:544–51, e1–7.

[95] Wambre E, Delong JH, James EA, Torres-Chinn N, Pfutzner W, Mobs C, et al. Specific immunotherapy modifies allergen-specific CD4(1) T-cell responses in an epitope-dependent manner. J Allergy Clin Immunol 2014;133:872–9.e7.with some proven efficacy clinically.

[96] Werfel T, Allam JP, Biedermann T, et al. Cellular and molecular immunologic mechanisms in patients with atopic dermatitis. J Allergy Clin Immunol. 2016;138(2):336–349. doi: 10.1016/j.jaci.2016.06.010.

[97] Brunner PM, Guttman-Yassky E, Leung DY. The immunology of atopic dermatitis and its reversibility with

broad-spectrum and targeted therapies. J Allergy Clin Immunol. 2017;139(4S): S65-S76. doi:10.1016/j.jaci.2017.01.011.

[98] Moyle M, Cevikbas F, Harden JL, Guttman-Yassky E. Understanding the immune landscape in atopic dermatitis: The era of biologics and emerging therapeutic approaches. Exp Dermatol. 2019;28(7):756–768. doi:10.1111/exd.13911.

[99] Abboud R, Choi J, Ruminski P, et al. Insights into the role of the JAK/STAT signaling pathway in graft-versus-host disease. Therapeutic Advances in Hematology. January 2020. doi:10.1177/2040620720914489

[100] Muraro A., Lemanske RF, Hellings PW., Akdis CA, Bieber T, Casale TB., et al. Precision medicine in patients with allergic diseases: Airway diseases and atopic dermatitis—PRACTALL document of the European Academy of Allergy and Clinical Immunology and the American Academy of Allergy, Asthma & Immunology. J Allergy Clin Immunol 2016;137:1347–58 http://dx.doi.org/10.1016/j.jaci.2016.03.010

[101] Eyerich S, Eyerich K, Pennino D, Carbone T, Nasorri F, Pallotta S, et al. Th22 cells represent a distinct human T cell subset involved in epidermal immunity and remodeling. J Clin Invest 2009;119:3573–85.

[102] Hijnen D, Knol EF, Gent YY, Giovannone B, Beijn SJ, Kupper TS, et al. CD8(1) T cells in the lesional skin of atopic dermatitis and psoriasis patients are an important source of IFN-gamma, IL-13, IL-17, and IL-22. J Invest Dermatol 2013; 133:973–9.

[103] Roesner LM, Heratizadeh A, Begemann G, Kienlin P, Hradetzky S, Niebuhr M, et al. Der p1 and Der p2-specific T cells display a Th2, Th17, and Th2/Th17 phenotype in atopic dermatitis. J Invest Dermatol 2015;135:2324–7.

[104] Bieber T. Stratified medicine: a new challenge for academia, industry, regulators and patients. London: Future Medicine; 2013; 75.

[105] Silverberg NB. A practical overview of pediatric atopic dermatitis, part 2: triggers and grading. Cutis. 2016; 97(5):326–329.

[106] Silverberg NB. A practical overview of pediatric atopic dermatitis, part 1: epidemiology and pathogenesis. Cutis. 2016;97(4):267–271.

[107] Handout on health: atopic dermatitis (a type of eczema). National Institute of Arthritis and Musculoskeletal and Skin Diseases website. https://www.niams.nih.gov/Health_Info/Atopic_Dermatitis/. Published July 2016. Accessed April 13, 2017

[108] Jaros J, Wilson C, Shi VY. Fabric Selection in Atopic Dermatitis: An Evidence-Based Review. Am J Clin Dermatol 21, 467–482 (2020). https://doi.org/10.1007/s40257-020-00516-0.

[109] Kanda N, Hoashi T, Saeki H. The Roles of Sex Hormones in the Course of Atopic Dermatitis. Int J Mol Sci 2019;20 (19):4660. Published 2019 Sep 20. doi: 10.3390/ijms20194660.

[110] Thestrup-Pedersen K, Ring J. Atopic dermatitis: Summary of the 1 Georg Rajka Symposium 1998and a literature review. Acta Derm Venereol. 1999;79:257–64. [PubMed: 10429979]

[111] Muluk NB, Altın F, Cingi C. Role of Superantigens in Allergic Inflammation: Their Relationship to Allergic Rhinitis, Chronic Rhinosinusitis, Asthma, and Atopic Dermatitis. Am J Rhinol Allergy. 2018;32(6):502–517. doi:10.1177/1945892418801083

[112] Tomczak H, Wróbel J, Jenerowicz D, et al. The role of *Staphylococcus aureus* in atopic

dermatitis: microbiological and immunological implications. Postepy Dermatol Alergol. 2019;36(4):485–491. doi:10.5114/ada.2018.77056. PMID: 31616226; PMCID: PMC6791154. 75

[113] Sun L, Liu W, Zang L. The Role of Toll-Like Receptors in Skin Host Defense, Psoriasis, and Atopic Dermatitis. J. Immunol. Res 201 9, Article ID 1824624, 13 pages. https://doi.org/10.1155/2019/1824624

[114] Leung DYM. New Insights into Atopic Dermatitis: Role of Skin Barrier and Immune Dysregulation New Insights into Atopic Dermatitis: Role of Skin Barrier and Immune Dysregulation. Allergol. Int 2013;62: 151–161. doi: 10.2332allergolint.13-RAI-0564.

[115] Damour A, Garcia M, Seneschal J, et al. Eczema Herpeticum: Clinical and Pathophysiological Aspects. Clinic Rev Allerg Immunol 2020;59:1–18. https://doi.org/10.1007/s12016-019-08768-3.

[116] Nguyen HLT, Trujillo-Paez JV, Umehara Y, Yue H, Peng G, Kiatsurayanon C, Chieosilapatham P, Song P, Okumura K, Ogawa H, Ikeda S, Niyonsaba F. Role of Antimicrobial Peptides in Skin Barrier Repair in Individuals with Atopic Dermatitis. Int. J. Mol. Sci. 2020; 21(20):7607. https://doi.org/10.3390/ijms21207607.

[117] Nowicka D, Grywalska E. The Role of Immune Defects and Colonization of *Staphylococcus aureus* in the Pathogenesis of Atopic Dermatitis. Anal. Cell. Pathol. May 2015;1–8. https://doTomczaki.org/10.1155/2018/1956403.

[118] Dickel H, Kuhlmann L, Bauer A, et al. H. Atopy patch testing with aeroallergens in a large clinical population of dermatitis patients in Germany and Switzerland, 2000–2015: a retrospective multicentre study. J. Eur. Acad. Dermatol. Venereol 2020;34: 2086–2095.

[119] Čelakovská J, Ettlerová K, Ettler K, Vaněčková J, Bukač J. Sensitization to aeroallergens in atopic dermatitis patients: association with concomitant allergic diseases. J Eur Acad Dermatol Venereol 2015;29(8):1500–1505. doi: 10.1111/jdv.12891

[120] Gutgesell C, Heise S, Seubert S, Seubert A, Domhof S, Brunner E, et al. Double-blind placebo-controlled house dust mite control measures in adult patients with atopic dermatitis. Br J Dermatol. 2001;145:70–4. doi:10.1046/j.1365-2133.2001.04283.x.

[121] Ghaderi R, Rashavi M. Prevalence of common allergens among patients with atopic dermatitis in Eastern Iran. MOJ Immunol 2018;6(3):74–80. DOI: 10.15406/moji.2018.06.00197

[122] Turnbull JL, Adams HN, Gorard DA. The diagnosis and management of food allergy and food intolerances. Aliment Pharmacol Ther 2015;41(1):3–25.

[123] Robison RG, Singh AM. Controversies in Allergy: Food Testing and Dietary Avoidance in Atopic Dermatitis. J Allergy Clin Immunol Pract 2019;7(1):35–39. doi:10.1016/j.jaip.2018.11.006]. 88

[124] Čelakovská J, Bukač J. Severity of atopic dermatitis in relation to food and inhalant allergy in adults and adolescents, Food Agr Immunol 2017;28 (1):121–133. doi: 10.1080/09540105.2016.1228838. 89

[125] Boye JI. Food allergies in developing and emerging economies: need for comprehensive data on prevalence rates. Clin Transl Allergy 2012;2:25. http://www.ctajournal.com/content/2/1/25

[126] Dhar S, Srinivas SM. Food Allergy in Atopic Dermatitis. Indian J Dermatol. 2016;61(6):645–648. doi:10.4103/0019-5154.193673 91

[127] Sugita K, Akdis CA. Recent developments and advances in atopic dermatitis and food allergy. Allergol Int 2020;69(2):204–214. https://doi.org/10.1016/j.alit.2019.08.013.

[128] Burks AW, Sampson HA, Plaut M, Lack G, Akdis CA. Treatment for food allergy. J Allergy Clin Immunol 2018; 141:1e9

[129] Liu P, Zhao Y, Mu ZL, Lu QJ, Zhang L, Yao X, Zheng M, Tang YW, Lu XX, Xia XJ, Lin YK, Li YZ, Tu CX, Yao ZR, Xu JH, Li W, Lai W, Yang HM, Xie HF, Han XP, Xie ZQ, Nong X, Guo ZP, Deng DQ, Shi TX, Zhang JZ. Clinical Features of Adult/Adolescent Atopic Dermatitis and Chinese Criteria for Atopic Dermatitis. Chin Med J 2016; 129:757–62

[130] Heli M, Aubert H, Bernier C, Néel A, Barbarot S. Atopic dermatitis of the adult. Rev Med Interne. 2016;37: 91–9.

[131] Silvestre Salvador JF, Romero-Pérez D, Encabo-Durán B. Atopic Dermatitis in Adults: A Diagnostic Challenge. J Investig Allergol Clin Immunol. 2017;27(2):78–88. DOI: 10.18176/jiaci.0138.

[132] Son JH, Chung BY, Kim HO, Park CW. Clinical Features of Atopic Dermatitis in Adults Are Different according to Onset. J Korean Med Sci. 2017;32(8):1360–1366. doi:10.3346/jkms.2017.32.8.1360

[133] Seghers AC, Lee JS, Tan CS, Koh YP, Ho MS, Lim YL, Giam YC, Tang MB. Atopic dirty neck or acquired atopic hyperpigmentation? An epidemiological and clinical study from the National Skin Centre in Singapore. Dermatology. 2014;229:174–82.

[134] Seghers AC, Lee JS, Tan CS, et al. Atopic dirty neck or acquired atopic hyperpigmentation? An epidemiological and clinical study from the National Skin Centre in Singapore. Dermatology 2014; 229(3):174–182. doi:10.1159/00036259699

[135] Kuriyama S, Kasuya A, Fujiyama T, Tatsuno K, Sakabe J, Yamaguchi H, Ito T, Tokura Y. Leukoderma in patients with atopic dermatitis. J Dermatol. 2015; 42:215–8.

[136] 2 Wollenberg A, Oranje A, Deleuran M, Simon D, Szalai Z, Kunz B, Svensson A, Barbarot S, von Kobyletzki L, Taieb A, de Bruin-Weller M, Werfel T, Trzeciak M, Vestergard C, Ring J, Darsow U; European Task Force on Atopic Dermatitis/EADV Eczema Task Force. ETFAD/EADV Eczema task force 2015 position paper on diagnosis and treatment of atopic dermatitis in adult and paediatric patients. J Eur Acad Dermatol Venereol. 2016:30;729–47.

[137] Grönhagen C, Liden C, Wahlgren C-F, Ballardini N, Bergström A, Kull I, Meding B. Hand eczema and atopic dermatitis in adolescents: a prospective cohort study from the BAMSE project. Br J Dermatol. 2015; 173:1175–82.

[138] Williams J, Cahill J, Nixon R. Occupational autoeczematization or atopic eczema precipitated by occupational contact dermatitis? Contact Dermatitis. 2007:56:21–6.

[139] Tanei R, Katsuoka K. Clinical analyses of atopic dermatitis in the aged. J Dermatol. 2008;35:562–569.

[140] Tanei R. Clinical characteristics, treatments, and prognosis of atopic eczema in the elderly. J Clin Med. 2015; 4:979–97.

[141] Oakley A. SCORAD – Codes and Concepts. DermNet NZ. Available at: https://dermnetnz.org/topics/scorad/ Used under the Creative Commons Licence http://creativecommons.org.nz/the-noncommercial-licences/

[142] Angelova-Fischer I, Bauer A, Hipler UC, et al. (October 2005). "The

objective severity assessment of atopic dermatitis (OSAAD) score: validity, reliability and sensitivity in adult patients with atopic dermatitis". Br. J. Dermatol. 153 (4): 767–73. doi:10.1111/j.1365-2133.2005.06697.x. PMID 16181458.

[143] "Severity scoring of atopic dermatitis: the SCORAD index. Consensus Report of the European Task Force on Atopic Dermatitis". Dermatology. 186 (1): 23–31. 1993. doi: 10.1159/000247298. PMID 8435513.

[144] SCORAD. Wikipedia. Available at: https://en.wikipedia.org/wiki/SCORAD. Accessed 11th December 2020.

[145] Wise F, Sulzberger MB. Editorial remarks, In The 1933 Year Book of Dermatology and Syphilology. Year Book Publishers Inc., Chicago, 1933;59.

[146] Hanifin JM, Rajka G. Diagnostic features of atopic dermatitis. Acta Derm Venereol Suppl (Stockh). 1980; 92:44–47.

[147] Williams H, Burney P, Pembroke A, Hay R. The U.K. Working Party's Diagnostic Criteria for Atopic Dermatitis. III. Independent hospital validation. Br. J. Dermatol. 1994;131: 406–416. DOI:10.1111/j.1365-2133.1994.tb08532.x

[148] Barrett M, Luu M. Differential Diagnosis of Atopic Dermatitis. Immunol Allergy Clin N Am. 2017;37 (1):11–34. DOI: 10.1016/j.iac.2016.08.009 PMID: 27886900.

[149] Sinclair W, Aboobaker J, Green RJ, Levin ME. Diagnosis of atopic dermatitis: From bedside to laboratory. S Afr Med. J 2014;104(10):711. DOI: 10.7196/SAMJ.8850.

[150] Segal, AO, Ellis, AK, Kim, HL. CSACI position statement: safety of topical calcineurin inhibitors in the management of atopic dermatitis in children and adults. Allergy Asthma Clin Immunol. 2013;9(1):24. doi: 10.1186/1710-1492-9-24.115

[151] Remitz A, De Pita O, Mota A, Serra-Baldrich E, Vakirlis E, Kapp A. Position statement: topical calcineurin inhibitors in atopic dermatitis. J Eur Acad Dermatol Venereol 2018;32:2074–2082. doi: 10.1111/jdv.15272.

[152] Ohtsuki, M, Morimoto, H, Nakagawa, H. Tacrolimus ointment for the treatment of adult and pediatric atopic dermatitis: review on safety and benefits. J Dermatol. 2018;45(8):936–942. doi:10.1111/1346-8138.14501

[153] Jarnagin K, Chanda S, Coronado D, et al. Crisaborole topical ointment, 2%: a nonsteroidal, topical, anti-inflammatory phosphodiesterase 4 inhibitor in clinical development for the treatment of atopic dermatitis. J Drugs Dermatol 2016; 15: 390–6. PubMed.

[154] Patrizi A, Raone B, Ravaioli GM. Management of atopic dermatitis: safety and efficacy of phototherapy. Clin Cosmet Investig Dermatol 2015;8:511–520. https://doi.org/10.2147/CCID.S87987.

[155] Ordóñez Rubiano MF, Arenas CM, Chalela JG. UVA-1 phototherapy for the management of atopic dermatitis: a large retrospective study conducted in a low-middle income country. Int J Dermatol 2018;57(7):799–803. doi: 10.1111/ijd.14011.

[156] Fernández-Guarino M, Aboin-Gonzalez S, Barchino L, Velazquez D, Arsuaga C, Lázaro P. Treatment of moderate and severe adult chronic atopic dermatitis with narrow-band UVB and the combination of narrow-band UVB/UVA phototherapy. Dermatol Ther 2016;29(1):19–23. doi: 10.1111/dth.12273.

[157] Megna M, Napolitano M, Patruno C, et al. Systemic Treatment of Adult Atopic Dermatitis: A Review.

Dermatol Ther (Heidelb) 2017;7:1–23. DOI 10.1007/s13555-016-0170-1.

[158] He A, Feldman SR, Fleischer AB Jr. An assessment of the use of antihistamines in the management of atopic dermatitis. J Am Acad Dermatol 2018;79(1):92–96. doi:10.1016/j.jaad.2017.12.077.

[159] Puterman A, Lewis H, Sinclair W, Green RJ. Topical and systemic pharmacological treatment of atopic dermatitis. S Afr Med J 2014 Aug;104 (10):714.

[160] Alfayi BA, Al-asiri SA, Al-Gelban LOS, et al. Efficiency and the adverse effect of systematic corticosteroid therapy for atopic dermatitis. J sci eng 2018;9(7):618–630.

[161] Drucker AM, Eyerich MS, de Bruin-Weller JP, et al. Use of systemic corticosteroids for atopic dermatitis: International Eczema Council consensus statement. Br J Dermatol 2018;178:768–775. doi: 10.1111/bjd.15928.

[162] Shah N, Alhusayen R, Walsh S, Shear NH. Methotrexate in the Treatment of Moderate to Severe Atopic Dermatitis: A Retrospective Study. J Cutan Med Surg. 2018;22(5):484–487. doi:10.1177/1203475418781336.

[163] Deleanu D, Nedelea I. Biological therapies for atopic dermatitis: An update (Review). Exp Ther Med 2019; 17: 1061–1067

[164] Montes-Torres A, Llamas-Velasco M, Pérez-Plaza A, Solano-López G, Sánchez-Pérez J. Biological Treatments in Atopic Dermatitis. J Clin Med 2015;4(4): 593–613. doi:10.3390/jcm4040593126

[165] Nygaard U, Vestergaard C, Deleuran, M. Systemic Treatment of Severe Atopic Dermatitis in Children and Adults. Curr Treat Options Allergy 2014;1:384–396. https://doi.org/10.1007/s40521-014-0032-y.128.

[166] Gooderham MJ, Hong HC, Eshtiaghi P, Papp KA. Dupilumab: A review of its use in the treatment of atopic dermatitis. J Am Acad Dermatol. 2018 Mar;78(3 Suppl 1): S28-S36. doi: 10.1016/j.jaad.2017.12.022. PMID: 29471919.

Chapter 6

Phototherapy in Atopic Dermatitis

Aleksandra Lesiak, Magdalena Ciazynska and Joanna Narbutt

Abstract

Atopic dermatitis (AD) is an inflammatory, recurrent and chronic disease that occurs in 2–10% of the population. Therapy of AD could be divided into topical (corticosteroids, calcineurin inhibitors) and systemic (cyclosporine, methotrexate, azathioprine or biological treatment). Phototherapy is taken into consideration as a second-line treatment, when topical therapy is unsuccessful. We distinguish many types of phototherapy, e.g. narrowband UVB (311–313 nm), UVA-1 therapy (340–400 nm), UVA/B combination, UVA therapy plus 8-methoxypsoralens (PUVA), 308 nm excimer laser (EL) and blue light. Phototherapy is effective in many cases, whether in adults or in children. It should be remembered that during therapy possible side effects may occur. Among them the risk of carcinogenesis is the most severe.

Keywords: atopic dermatitis, phototherapy, eczema, NB-UVB therapy, UVA-1 therapy PUVA therapy, blue light

1. Introduction

Atopy refers to a personal tendency to heightened immune responses to small doses of allergens and as a result producing IgE antibodies. As a consequence a patient develops certain types of diseases, such as atopic dermatitis, allergic rhinitis and asthma.

Atopic dermatitis (AD) is a dermatosis that occurs in 2–5% of the population and is one of the most common dermatoses. Nowadays in developed countries over the past three decades the number of cases of AD has almost tripled. The main symptoms of the disease are pruritis, abnormally dry skin and erythema. Atopic dermatitis is characterized by chronic or relapsing course. The onset of AD in most cases is observed during early childhood. In infants, lesions appear mostly on cheeks and extremities, whereas in children and adults – in flexural areas. The lesions are combined with hyperkeratosis and lichenification. Triggering factors such as stress, wool intolerance or sweating may worsen the course of AD. During therapy avoiding those is highly desirable. *Staphylococcus aureus* is one of the microorganisms which can be found on the skin of AD patients. It is present not only on erythematous lesions, but also on a "healthy" skin.

The first line of AD therapy is a short-term regimen – when the patient uses medicines only when inflammatory lesions occur, but in recent years the therapy is more focused on proactive and long-term maintenance. Drugs should be applied continuously or one/two times a week. The basic rule in the therapy is to use emollients which restore epidermal barrier and create an occluding coating. Therefore, they protect the skin from triggering factors. In mild course of AD using topical corticosteroids and topical calcineurin inhibitors is recommended. In moderate to severe cases of AD phototherapy, cyclosporine, methotrexate, azathioprine or systemic corticosteroids may be administered. Phototherapy (using ultraviolet light) is also useful in other inflammatory skin diseases, like psoriasis. We distinguish the following types of phototherapy:

- broadband UVB (290–320 nm),
- narrowband UVB (311–313 nm),
- UVA-1 therapy (340–400 nm),
- UVA therapy plus 8-methoxypsoralens (PUVA),
- 308 nm excimer laser (EL),
- blue light (BL).

2. Mechanism of action

Phototherapy (specifically broadband UVB) in atopic dermatitis has been used since 1970 and its effectiveness is clinically proven [1]. The mechanism of skin lesions development in atopic dermatitis is connected with activation of T-cell infiltration into the skin, which leads to increasing proliferation of keratinocytes and as a result thickening of the skin. Th2 cells accumulate and produce various cytokines, such as IL-4, IL-31, IL-13. Th1 cells, INF- γ, Th22 cells and IL-22 were also found in chronic atopic lesions [2]. Common type of drugs used in AD are immunosuppressants. We divide them into systemic (cyclosporine) and topical (tacrolimus, pimecrolimus) types. They act by inhibiting calcineurin which leads to a decrease in activation of T cells. It indicates that targeting T cells may be an effective approach in therapy of AD.

Artificial or natural ultraviolet radiation leads to deep immunosuppression which induces apoptic death in activated T cells. Many factors, such as wavelength, dosage of radiation, amount of UV sessions have an impact on the intensity of immunosuppressive effect of UV radiation. In general UV radiation could be dived into UVB (with wavelength between 280 and 320 nm) and UVA (with wavelength between 320 and 400 nm). Overall UVB light has a higher immunosuppressive impact than UVA. Psoralens in PUVA therapy are molecules whose purpose is intercalation of DNA. After UVA radiation psoralens are binding to the DNA. This results in stopping cells proliferation [3]. Nowadays more and more diseases are treated with biological therapy. Owing to good safety profile, accessibility, only topical immunosuppression and cost-effectiveness of UV radiation, phototherapy is still a very popular AD therapy. Biological effects of UV radiation are complex and could be classified into instantaneous and delayed [4]. Damage of DNA and cytoplasmic membrane, induction of cytoplasmic transcriptional factors and chromophore's isomerization initiates immediate stunted growth and, as a consequence, apoptosis [5].

After UVB radiation, photon's absorption causes changes of DNA molecular structures. As a result, transcription of DNA is paused and cell cycle in fibroblasts and epidermal cells stops (phototype I reaction) [6]. In PUVA phototherapy after psoralen application with following UVA radiation, reactive oxygen species are damaging DNA and cell membrane (phototype II reaction) [7]. After only one hour DNA starts to repair and the cells start to proliferate. As an effect in 48–72 hours after UV radiation short-term effects are reversing. Long term effects refer to inhibition of immune cells which causes immunosuppression. Induction of apoptosis in epidermal and dermal T cells is a crucial mechanism [8]. Apoptosis after UVB radiation concerns keratinocytes too, leading to lesions clearance. Moreover, UVB and PUVA activate T regulatory (Treg) cells and decrease the amount of presenting antigen in Langerhans cells [9].

After UV radiation cytokine secretion and number of macrophages are limited. Acting through reactive oxygen species, neutrophils and NK cells are suppressed [10]. As an effect cytokine balance is changed – decrease of inflammatory cytokines IL-2, IL-8, IL-9, IL-17, IL-22, IL-23, TNF-a and IFN- γ with simultaneous induction of immunosuppressive cytokine – IL-10 [11].

3. Types

3.1 NB-UVB

NB UV-B has been in use of AD treatment since 1990 [28]. It emits highly selective UV-B light wavelengths (from 311 to 313 nm, without shortwave length UVB) [12]. Sunburning potential of NB UV-B is evidently lower than broadband UV-B (BB UV-B) [13]. Due to the long list of advantages, like safety profile, effectiveness, accessibility NB UV-B could be pondered as a first-line treatment [14]. It has been established in many randomized trials that NB-UVB therapy improved the scores of AD and the necessity for applying potent topical corticosteroids was reduced [15]. These type of positive results remained up to six months after the scheme of NB-UVB was finished [16]. Contrary to UVA, NB UV-B does not penetrate the dermis, therefore it is limited to the epidermis [15]. Patient's tolerance to UV radiation and pigmentation of the skin determines the dosage of UV-B. When it comes to the methods of adjusting UV-B dose which should be administered, the most popular is defining "Minimal Erythema Dose" (MED). MED refers to the smallest UV-B dose which is capable of provoking minimal erythema on the patient's skin [17]. Skin phototype can play a role in determining UV-B dosage. Measuring skin reflectance is another way of UV-B dose calculation and it was derived from defining the skin pigmentation. It is called reflectance-guided UV-B and recently it has become highly popular [18]. Most physicians use NB UV-B treatment schedule which consists of three sessions of radiation every six weeks [19]. In early studies, researchers used nearly erythemogenic dose of NB UV-B, but recently it was proven, that reducing a dose by half can give similar outcome, higher tolerance and lower risk of carcinogenesis. Reports comparing UV-A1 and NB-UVB are ambivalent [15]. Some of them point to superiority of NB UV-B, other do not show statistically significant differences [20]. In some cases NB UV-B can be combined with UV-A1 in one therapy schedule with satisfying clinical effect [21].

In literature there is strong evidence proving efficacy of AD therapy using NB-UVB. In a study with a test group of 21 adults with severe course of the disease, administering air-conditioned NB-UVB thrice a week for twelve weeks caused reduction of severity (68%) and reduction of topical corticosteroid application (88%). 15 of 21 patients showed positive result 24 weeks after therapy ended [12]. Brazzelli et al. in their study reported efficacy of treating AD with NB UV-B, proceeded by oral short-term cyclosporin A (four weeks) and four-six-week-long washout phase. Radiation was administered three times a week and lasted up to two months [22]. There were some studies concerning NB UV-B therapy of atopic dermatitis in children. Jury et al. in their retrospective trial on 25 children with AD showed almost total reduction of lesions in 17 patients [23]. NB-UVB is a recommended therapeutic option in pregnancy [24].

Prospective clinical trial with 29 children (3–16 years old) pointed 61% reduction in SASSAD score (Six Area Six Sign Atopis Dermatitis) in a group exposed to NB UV-B radiation in comparison to untreated patients ($P < 0.05$). Moreover, children without therapy experienced a decrease in the quality of life with a rise of disease severity [25].

3.2 UVA1

Development of UVA1 (340-400 nm) lamps was a response to appearing side effects, such as long exposure time or risk of sunburn when using UVA-2 (320-340 nm) radiation. UVA-1 penetrates deeper into the dermis than UVA-2 and UVB [26]. We distinguish different types of doses:

- high dose (80–130 J/cm^2),
- medium dose (40–80 J/cm^2)
- low dose (<40 J/cm^2) [27, 28].

It should be mentioned that a huge inconvenience of UV-A1 in high dose is overheating of the device, which can be unsafe. Studies showed that UV-A1 is more efficient in AD therapy and has higher efficacy than UV-AB. Krutmann et all proved that UV-A1 phototherapy effectiveness is approximately the same as therapy with fluocortolone [28]. Medium doses of UVA-A1 have the advantage over high doses of UVA-A1 when it comes to reducing adverse drug events and enhancing tolerance. The effectiveness and relapse time do not differ strongly between these two options of therapy. Therefore the UVA-A1 radiation should be the preferable one [1]. UVA-A1 in low doses is practically ineffective, thereby it is not considered to be a therapeutic agent [28]. Common treatment schedules of UVA-A1 at medium dose (maximum 80 J/cm2) in atopic dermatitis therapy are 3–5 sessions every 3–8 weeks. Patient should spend 10 minutes to 1 hour in every phototherapy session [15, 29]. Speaking of acute cases of AD, using UV-A1 radiation is more suitable, comparing to UV-B [15]. Majoie et al. examined 13 adults (20–56 years old) suffering from chronic atopic dermatitis in a randomized investigator-blinded trial and proved that NB-UVB and medium dose of UVA1 are comparably efficient in the reduction of AD symptoms [20]. The disadvantage of UV-A1 therapy is the cost and the size of UV-A1 lamps. Moreover, they demand a presence of ventilation machines, what could be financially unachievable for some centers [30]. To meet the expectations of the patients engineers created a filter to eliminate wavelengths above 530 nm and disperse the excessive heat. It is called Cold-light UV-A1 and it is consider a more effective option than UV-AB and classic UV-A1 in treatment of AD flares [31].

3.3 PUVA

PUVA (psoralen and ultraviolet A) is a combination of UVA light and psoralens – a substance causing photosensitizing effect. Nowadays in use there is an 8-methoxypsoralen (8-MOP), which leads to permanent damage of DNA [13]. Psoralens are available in many various formulations, such as pills, cream or bath lotion [32]. In bath-PUVA, the patient is taking a bath in warm water with 8-MOP 20–30 minutes before UVA session. In case of choosing cream formulation, the regimen is conducted

30–60 minutes before radiation [32]. Using topical psoralens could be desired, for example in patients with strictly localized lesions. In literature it is proven that PUVA phototherapy could be a successful form of atopic dermatitis therapy [33]. Although, we should remember that in comparison with other inflammatory diseases treated by PUVA, in atopic dermatitis patients require more phototherapy sessions [15]. Der-Petrossian M. et al. in a randomized trial compared PUVA bath therapy with NB UV-B – there were no significant differences between these types of phototherapy [33]. In another study Tzaneva S. et al. showed that after PUVA therapy (using oral 5-methoxypsoralen, 5-MOP) patients had longer remission times and higher change in AD scoring compared to UV-A1 phototherapy [34]. Heinlin et al., in his randomized and placebo-controlled trial demonstrated superiority of balneophototherapy and NB-UVB combination over only NB-UVB. Patients' complex therapy had higher reduction of SCORAD score not only at the end of treatment, but also after 6 months. (P respectively <0,004 and < 0,04) [16]. Because of mutagenic properties of PUVA therapy, it should be reminded that it could not be a chronic form of therapy and using it should be limited [30].

3.4 UVA/B combination

UVA and UVA combination (280-400 nm) can be conducted by using special machines emitting these UV spectrums or as two separate sessions. In clinical trial Valkova and Velkova proved that combination UVA/B phototherapy with topical corticosteroids reduced the treatment duration significantly in comparison to only UVA/B (P = 0.02) [35]. Grandulad et al. investigated reduction of SCORAD, days in remission and the improvement in quality of life using ciclosporin and UVA/B. Ciclosporin had statistically significantly better scores compared to UVA/B phototherapy sessions [36]. Jekler [37] and Larko [38] showed that using the combination of UVA/B radiation is more effective than monotherapy of UVA or UVB.

3.5 Excimer laser

Monochromatic excimer laser (MEL) is a kind of single-wavelength light source of 308 nm. The advantage of this therapy is a frequency of sessions – every 7–15 days [39]. MEL could be used on the localized skin lesions. One study showed good ability of alleviation of prurigo in AD. However, further clinical trials are needed [40].

3.6 Blue light

Blue light (400-495 nm) is a novel therapeutic option. Becker et al. in his observational study showed that using blue light devices could the suitable in treatment severe atopic dermatitis. In addition, it provided to long term improvement. Observed adverse effects were mild and transient – redness, warmth or itching the skin. [41] Kromer et al. is performing a multicenter, prospective randomized, placebo controlled, double blinded trial with 150 patients suffering from AD to investigate effectiveness of blue light devices. Currently there are no official results, but that investigation appears to be promising [42].

4. Side effects

Like every therapeutic agent, phototherapy may cause some side effects. Most of them are mild and short-term, for example skin burning (connected with wrong dosage of UV or inadequate radiation schedule), pruritus, hyperpigmentation, dryness and tenderness. Induction of polymorphic light eruptions and viruses reinfection (such a herpes simplex) are also observed. When it comes to long-term adverse effects, photo-aging and induction of cutaneous malignancies can occur [14]. These cutaneous malignances can be caused by combing UV radiation with other therapeutic factors. There is a reported case of a melanoma diagnosis in a patient with mastocytosis who was treated with UVA1 and PUVA bath therapy previously [42]. In literature we can find two cases of Merkel cell carcinoma after UVA1 therapy in patients who were treated with immunosuppressants for blood dyscrasias [43].

Lately new therapeutic options were presented. One of them is 308 nm monochromatic excimer light. It is dedicated for patients with localized and therapy-resistant lesions [44]. In comparison to other immunosuppressive agents, phototherapy has a better safety profile, adverse effects are milder and better-tolerated [23]. PUVA systemic therapy can cause hepatotoxicity, nausea, vomiting, cataract, long-term photosensitivity and probable skin cancer. Topical use of psoralens can limit or help avoid these inconveniences [45]. However, please note that atopic dermatitis is a chronic and recurrent disease which implicates many phototherapy sessions and increases the risk of carcinogenesis [16]. Many clinical trials showed that phototherapy in children with AD is effective and, in most cases, well tolerated. There is, nonetheless, high risk of photocarcinogenesis. In younger patients long-term maintenance therapy should be conducted in as short time as possible [23]. In conclusion, this way of AD treatment is one of the last therapeutic options. Claustrophobia and lack of cooperation is typical for small children and it has to be taken into consideration as a challenge in this kind of therapy [15]. Despite this, in children with refractory or severe atopic dermatitis we may consider using phototherapy. Generally, in such cases, NB UV-B is a therapy of choice and PUVA should be avoided [23]. It should be also remembered that there are no randomized trials of phototherapy of AD in pregnancy [30]. UV treatment require specific amount of time and availability, which can be problematic for patients who are attending school or have strict work hours. To meet these demands, there are some home phototherapy devices accessible.

5. Conclusions

Phototherapy is considered as a safe and successful therapy in management of atopic dermatitis. When topical corticosteroids and calcineurin inhibitors are ineffective, phototherapy could be considered as a second line treatment, whether in combination with systemic drugs or without them. The most effective types of phototherapy are UVA1 and NB-UVB; UVA1 should be pondered in acute flares whereas NB-UVB in recurrent atopic dermatitis. In children and pregnancy NB-UVB has a good safety profile. Using UVA1 medium dose of radiation has an advantage over others. Due to safety profile narrow-band UVB is favored over broad-band UVB. Potential adverse effects are usually mild and transient, although the risk of carcinogenesis should be always considered.

DOI: http://dx.doi.org/10.5772/intechopen.94215

Author details

Aleksandra Lesiak[1*], Magdalena Ciazynska[2] and Joanna Narbutt[1]

1 Department of Dermatology, Pediatric Dermatology and Oncology, Medical University of Lodz, Lodz, Poland

2 Dermoklinika Centrum Medyczne, Lodz, Poland

*Address all correspondence to: lesiak_ola@interia.pl

References

[1] A. Pérez-Ferriols et al., "Modalidades de fototerapia para el tratamiento de la dermatitis atópica: revisión sistemática de la literatura," *Actas Dermosifiliogr.*, vol. 106, no. 5, pp. 387-401, Jun. 2015.

[2] R. Sabat, K. Wolk, L. Loyal, W. D. Döcke, and K. Ghoreschi, "T cell pathology in skin inflammation," *Seminars in Immunopathology*, vol. 41, no. 3. Springer Verlag, pp. 359-377, 01-May-2019.

[3] F. A. Derheimer, J. K. Hicks, M. T. Paulsen, C. E. Canman, and M. Ljungman, "Psoralen-Induced DNA interstrand cross-links block transcription and induce p53 in an ataxia-telangiectasia and rad3-related-dependent manner," *Mol. Pharmacol.*, vol. 75, no. 3, pp. 599-607, Mar. 2009.

[4] T. Kopp, F. Karlhofer, Z. Szepfalusi, A. Schneeberger, G. Stingl, and A. Tanew, "Successful use of acitretin in conjunction with narrowband ultraviolet B phototherapy in a child with severe pustular psoriasis, von Zumbusch type," *Br. J. Dermatol.*, vol. 151, no. 4, pp. 912-916, Oct. 2004.

[5] M. S. Duthie, I. Kimber, and M. Norval, "The effects of ultraviolet radiation on the human immune system," *British Journal of Dermatology*, vol. 140, no. 6. Br J Dermatol, pp. 995-1009, 1999.

[6] H. P. Baden, J. M. Parrington, J. D. A. Delhanty, and M. A. Pathak, "DNA synthesis in normal and xeroderma pigmentosum fibroblasts following treatment with 8-methoxypsoralen and long wave ultraviolet light," *BBA Sect. Nucleic Acids Protein Synth.*, vol. 262, no. 3, pp. 247-255, Mar. 1972.

[7] J. Wenk *et al.*, "UV-induced oxidative stress and photoaging.," *Current problems in dermatology*, vol. 29. Curr Probl Dermatol, pp. 83-94, 2001.

[8] N. Schade, C. Esser, and J. Krutmann, "Ultraviolet B radiation-induced immunosuppression: Molecular mechanisms and cellular alterations," *Photochem. Photobiol. Sci.*, vol. 4, no. 9, pp. 699-708, Aug. 2005.

[9] F. Aubin and C. Mousson, "Ultraviolet light-induced regulatory (suppressor) T cells: An approach for promoting induction of operational allograft tolerance?," in *Transplantation*, 2004, vol. 77, no. 1 SUPPL.

[10] M. L. Weitzen and B. Bonavida, "Mechanism of inhibition of human natural killer activity by ultraviolet radiation.," *J. Immunol.*, vol. 133, no. 6, 1984.

[11] T. P. Singh *et al.*, " 8-Methoxypsoralen Plus Ultraviolet A Therapy Acts via Inhibition of the IL-23/Th17 Axis and Induction of Foxp3 + Regulatory T Cells Involving CTLA4 Signaling in a Psoriasis-Like Skin Disorder ," *J. Immunol.*, vol. 184, no. 12, pp. 7257-7267, Jun. 2010.

[12] S. A. George, D. J. Bilsland, B. E. Johnson, and J. Ferguson, "Narrow-band (TL-01) UVB air-conditioned phototherapy for chronic severe adult atopic dermatitis," *Br. J. Dermatol.*, vol. 128, no. 1, pp. 49-56, 1993.

[13] J. M. Carrascosa *et al.*, "Documento de consenso sobre fototerapia: Terapias PUVA y UVB de banda estrecha," *Actas Dermo-Sifiliograficas*, vol. 96, no. 10. Ediciones Doyma, S.L., pp. 635-658, 2005.

[14] D. L. Rodenbeck, J. I. Silverberg, and N. B. Silverberg, "Phototherapy for atopic dermatitis," *Clin. Dermatol.*, vol. 34, no. 5, pp. 607-613, 2016.

[15] N. B. Meduri, T. Vandergriff, H. Rasmussen, and H. Jacobe, "Phototherapy in the management of atopic dermatitis: A systematic review," *Photodermatology Photoimmunology and Photomedicine*, vol. 23, no. 4. Photodermatol Photoimmunol Photomed, pp. 106-112, Aug-2007.

[16] J. Heinlin *et al.*, "A first prospective randomized controlled trial on the efficacy and safety of synchronous balneophototherapy vs. narrow-band UVB monotherapy for atopic dermatitis," *J. Eur. Acad. Dermatology Venereol.*, vol. 25, no. 7, pp. 765-773, Jul. 2011.

[17] A. Pérez-Ferriols, "Proyecto dosis eritematosa mínima (DEM): en busca del consenso en la técnica del fototest," *Actas Dermosifiliogr.*, vol. 104, no. 7, pp. 541-542, Sep. 2013.

[18] E. Selvaag, L. Caspersen, N. Bech-Thomsen, and H. C. Wulf, "Optimized UVB treatment of atopic dermatitis using skin reflectance measurements. A controlled, left-right comparison trial," *Acta Derm. Venereol.*, vol. 85, no. 2, pp. 144-146, 2005.

[19] N. J. Reynolds, V. Franklin, J. C. Gray, B. L. Diffey, and P. M. Farr, "Narrow-band ultraviolet B and broad-band ultraviolet A phototherapy in adult atopic eczema: A randomised controlled trial," *Lancet*, vol. 357, no. 9273, pp. 2012-2016, Jun. 2001.

[20] I. M. L. Majoie *et al.*, "Narrowband ultraviolet B and medium-dose ultraviolet A1 are equally effective in the treatment of moderate to severe atopic dermatitis," *J. Am. Acad. Dermatol.*, vol. 60, no. 1, pp. 77-84, Jan. 2009.

[21] M. Fernández-Guarino, S. Aboin-Gonzalez, L. Barchino, D. Velazquez, C. Arsuaga, and P. Lázaro, "Treatment of moderate and severe adult chronic atopic dermatitis with narrow-band UVB and the combination of narrow-band UVB/UVA phototherapy," *Dermatol. Ther.*, vol. 29, no. 1, pp. 19-23, Jan. 2016.

[22] V. Brazzelli, F. Prestinari, M. G. Chiesa, R. G. Borroni, M. Ardigò, and G. Borroni, "Sequential treatment of severe atopic dermatitis with cyclosporin a and low-dose narrow-band UVB phototherapy [2]," *Dermatology*, vol. 204, no. 3. Dermatology, pp. 252-254, 2002.

[23] C. S. Jury, P. McHenry, A. D. Burden, R. Lever, and D. Bilsland, "Narrowband ultraviolet B (UVB) phototherapy in children," *Clin. Exp. Dermatol.*, vol. 31, no. 2, pp. 196-199, Mar. 2006.

[24] W. Placek *et al.*, "Phototherapy and photochemotherapy in dermatology. Recommendations of the Polish Dermatological Society," *Przegl. Dermatol.*, vol. 106, no. 3, pp. 237-256, 2019.

[25] E. Tan, D. Lim, and M. Rademaker, "Narrowband UVB phototherapy in children: A New Zealand experience," *Australas. J. Dermatol.*, vol. 51, no. 4, pp. 268-273, Nov. 2010.

[26] S. Attili, R. Dawe, and S. Ibbotson, "Ultraviolet A1 phototherapy: One center's experience," *Indian J. Dermatology, Venereol. Leprol.*, vol. 83, no. 1, p. 60, Jan. 2017.

[27] T. Diepgen, W. Czech, R. Niedner, A. Kapp, and E. Schöpf, "High-dose UVA1 therapy in the treatment of patients with atopic dermatitis," *J. Am. Acad. Dermatol.*, vol. 26, no. 2, pp. 225-230, 1992.

[28] J. Krutmann *et al.*, "High-dose UVA1 therapy for atopic dermatitis: Results of a multicenter trial," *J. Am. Acad. Dermatol.*, vol. 38, no. 4, pp. 589-593, 1998.

[29] S. Tzaneva, A. Seeber, M. Schwaiger, H. Hönigsmann, and A. Tanew, "High-dose versus medium-dose UVA1 phototherapy for patients with severe generalized atopic dermatitis," *J. Am. Acad. Dermatol.*, vol. 45, no. 4, pp. 503-507, 2001.

[30] A. Patrizi, B. Raone, and G. M. Ravaioli, "Management of atopic dermatitis: Safety and efficacy of phototherapy," *Clinical, Cosmetic and Investigational Dermatology*, vol. 8. Dove Medical Press Ltd., pp. 511-520, 05-Oct-2015.

[31] G. Von Kobyletzki, C. Pieck, K. Hoffmann, M. Freitag, and P. Altmeyer, "Medium-dose UVA1 cold-light phototherapy the treatment of severe atopic dermatitis," *J. Am. Acad. Dermatol.*, vol. 41, no. 6, pp. 931-937, 1999.

[32] W. L. MORISON, J. A. PARRISH, and T. B. FITZPATRICK, "Oral psoralen photochemotherapy of atopic eczema," *Br. J. Dermatol.*, vol. 98, no. 1, pp. 25-30, 1978.

[33] M. Der-Petrossian, A. Seeber, H. Hönigsmann, and A. Tanew, "Half-side comparison study on the efficacy of 8-methoxypsoralen bath- PUVA versus narrow-band ultraviolet B phototherapy in patients with severe chronic atopic dermatitis," *Br. J. Dermatol.*, vol. 142, no. 1, pp. 39-43, 2000.

[34] S. Tzaneva *et al.*, "5-Methoxypsoralen plus ultraviolet (UV) A is superior to medium-dose UVA1 in the treatment of severe atopic dermatitis: A randomized crossover trial," *Br. J. Dermatol.*, vol. 162, no. 3, pp. 655-660, 2010.

[35] S. Valkova and A. Velkova, "UVA/UVB phototherapy for atopic dermatitis revisited," *J. Dermatolog. Treat.*, vol. 15, no. 4, pp. 239-244, 2004.

[36] H. Granlund, Pekka Erkko, Anita Remitz, "Comparison of Cyclosporin and UVAB Phototherapy for Intermittent One-year Treatment of Atopic Dermatitis," *Acta Derm. Venereol.*, vol. 81, no. 1, pp. 22-27, Jan. 2001

[37] J. Jekler and O. Larkö, "Combined UVA-UVB versus UVB phototherapy for atopic dermatitis: A paired-comparison study," *J. Am. Acad. Dermatol.*, vol. 22, no. 1, pp. 49-53, Jan. 1990.

[38] J. O. Jekler Larko, "Phototherapy for atopic dermatitis with ultraviolet A (UVA), low-dose UVB and combined UVA and UVB: Two paired-comparison studies," *Photodermatol. Photoimmunol. Photomed.*, vol. 8, no. 4, pp. 151-156, Aug. 1991.

[39] L. Mavilia, M. Mori, *R. Rossi*, P. Campolmi, A. P. Guerra, and T. Lotti, "308 nm monochromatic excimer light in dermatology: personal experience and review of the literature.," *undefined*, 2008.

[40] E. E. A. Brenninkmeijer, P. I. Spuls, R. Lindeboom, A. C. Van Der Wal, J. D. Bos, and A. Wolkerstorfer, "Excimer laser vs. clobetasol propionate 0·05% ointment in prurigo form of atopic dermatitis: A randomized controlled trial, a pilot," *Br. J. Dermatol.*, vol. 163, no. 4, pp. 823-831, Oct. 2010.

[41] D. Becker *et al.*, "Clinical efficacy of blue light full body irradiation as treatment option for severe atopic dermatitis," *PLoS One*, vol. 6, no. 6, pp. 1-9, 2011.

[42] C. Kromer *et al.*, "Treatment of atopic dermatitis using a full-body blue light device (AD-BLUE): Protocol of a randomized controlled trial," *J. Med. Internet Res.*, vol. 21, no. 1, Jan. 2019.

[43] F. Trautinger, "Phototherapy of mycosis fungoides," *Photodermatol. Photoimmunol. Photomed.*, vol. 27, no. 2, pp. 68-74, Apr. 2011.

[44] R. C. Gathers, L. Scherschun, F. Malick, D. P. Fivenson, and H. W. Lim, "Narrowband UVB phototherapy for early-stage mycosis fungoides," *J. Am. Acad. Dermatol.*, vol. 47, no. 2, pp. 191-197, Aug. 2002.

[45] I. Wollenschläger, J. Hermann, and H. M. Ockenfels, "UVB-308-nm-(NUVB-)Therapie mittels Excimer-Laser bei atopischer Dermatitis und weiteren inflammatorischen Dermatosen," *Hautarzt*, vol. 60, no. 11, pp. 898-906, Nov. 2009.

Chapter 7

Probiotics in Allergic Diseases

Ivana Filipovic, Milan Lackovic, Slađana Mihajlovic, Đorđe Filipović, Tamara Bakic and Zorica Zivkovic

Abstract

Allergic diseases are the most common chronic diseases in children and no complete agreement on effective measures for primary prevention is available. Atopic family history is one of the most important risk factors for the development of asthma. A decline in microbial diversity due to modern lifestyle particularly in urban areas was proposed to have an important role in allergic epidemic. Recent studies are more focused on the specific mode of prevention such as probiotic usage in early pregnancy and infants period. It is well known that the composition of the gastrointestinal microbiota has been postulated to play a role in the development of allergies because it promotes potentially antiallergenic processes: TH1-type immunity, generation of TGF (which has an essential role in suppression of TH2-induced allergic inflammation and induction of oral tolerance), and IgA production, an essential component of mucosal immune defenses. Probiotic interventions administered during pregnancy and breastfeeding offer a unique opportunity to influence a range of important maternal and infant outcomes.

Keywords: allergy, atopic dermatitis, probiotics

1. Introduction

According to the epidemiological data, half of pediatric population will suffer from allergic diseases until the end of 2020. With that prevalence of more than 30%, they represent the most common disorders of children, adolescents, and adults [1]. A great increase of the prevalence of allergic diseases globally in the last 10 years are best described in a concept of “allergic epidemic” [2]. Germany multi-center allergy study is one of the most important epidemiological studies on allergic diseases, showing age related manifestation of allergic diseases, best described in “allergic march” concept. Allergies start in early infancy as an atopic dermatitis or food allergies, followed with the development of respiratory allergies such as allergic rhinitis and/or asthma [3]. Different from all other chronic diseases such as diabetes mellitus, hypertension, etc., allergic diseases manifest as it has been previously mentioned early in infancy, according to some authors even prenatal. It is well known that allergic diseases are multifactorial, so both environmental and genetic factors may play an important role in their pathogenesis. Identification of prenatal and early postnatal factors is of a great importance for early prevention and intervention [4–6]. Due to many phenotypes and genotypes as well as different patients’ needs although a great availability of pharmacological options, treating allergies still represents a great challenge. Detection of individual risk factors and identification of predictive markers are of a great importance in primary prevention, early intervention, and immune modulation of a natural course of allergic diseases [7]. It is well know that the development of immune system starts in 11 gestation week with the production of IgE antibodies. Detection of specific IgE antibodies on inhalatory and nutritive allergens is not possible in cord core blood. Except dry skin other clinical manifestation of allergies is not presented in infants. Atopic dermatitis will develop in the first year of life in a case of a great transdermal water loss between 2nd day of life and 2nd month of life. As we have already mentioned, both genetic and "in utero" environmental factors are responsible for allergy development. Uni or bilateral positive family history of allergies, diet habits, obesity, smoking, and drug use during pregnancy, season at time of birth as well as gestational age, the way of delivery are known to be an very important risk factors. Primary prevention and early intervention can prevent the development of atopic march. It includes treating skin with emollient creams, breast feeding in the first year of life, probiotics, and vitamin D during pregnancy and during the first year of life, early introduction of solid food as well as allergens [8]. Many hypotheses on causes of the increase in allergic diseases have been suggested. One of the most investigated hypotheses is "hygiene hypothesis", helping us to understand early-life events. It is well known that early exposure to common bacterial triggers such as endotoxins, LPS, or hemlines might have an allergy preventive effect.

The second worldwide accepted concept of reduced exposure (exposure to small amounts of foreign proteins) in exclusively breastfeeding children may rather lead to tolerance than to clinical allergic disease. Other routes of exposure via inhalation or via the skin cannot be totally avoided; interventional studies on avoidance/reduction of indoor allergen exposure (house dust mite and cat) have not shown convincing results. EAACI evidence-based recommendation for prevention of food and respiratory allergy prevention includes: no special diet during pregnancy or for the lactating mother, exclusively breastfeeding for 4–6 months, if needed hypoallergenic formula is recommended, avoids exposure to tobacco smoke, and avoids pets at home [9, 10].

2. The role of microbiome

All plants, animals, and humans live in close association with microbial organisms. The Human Microbiome Project has showed that the human body contains trillions of microorganisms which outnumber human cells by 10 to 1. Their genes encoded proteins essential for human survival. The role of microbes is of particular importance in gastrointestinal tract where they are involved in break down proteins, lipides, and carbohydrates in monomers suitable for absorption [11]. They are also involved in vitamin synthesis as well as in immuno modulation. Mice raised under germ free conditions have suffered from deficit in innate and adaptive immunity suggesting that the microbiome may play a crucial role in maturation of child immune system. Furthermore, experimental studies in germ free mice showed that those mice developed easily allergic diseases. Reconstruction of neonate mice with a conventional microbic protected the animals from allergic diseases.

The protective role of exposure to a wide diversity of microbial is best described in children raised on traditional farms [12]. Those children have a much lower prevalence of asthma, have fever, and allergic sensitization in comparison to children grown up in urban areas expect those who are exposed to environmental microbes (those who keep dogs indoors) [13].

Gut microbiota is one of the most investigated topics in the last couple of years. Human microbiota represent a community of commensal, symbiotic, and pathogenic bacteria that live in and on human body with the widest and probably most important community in human gut.

3. History of probiotics

Several thousand years ago, ancient Roman scientist Gaius Plinius Secundus Maior recommended fermented milk to treat gastrointestinal problems. Benefits of probiotics contained in sour milk cream or yogurt are mentioned even in Holy Bible. In 1900, Moro isolated the first bacteria that produced lactic acid Bacillus acidophilus later called Lactobacillus acidophilus. Ilja Iljic Mecnikov was the first scientist who proved benefits of so-called good lactic acid produced bacteria particularly on gastrointestinal tract. In his hypothesis on autointoxication, he claimed that human body is intoxicated with toxins and pathogenic bacteria from food and he proposed consumption of lactic acid bacteria contained in Bulgarian yogurt in treating this disorder. The bacteria isolated from Bulgarian yogurt later became famous under name Lactobacillus delbrueckii strain, substring bulgaricus.

Henri Tiser from Pasteur Institute isolated Bifidobacterium bifidum from the feces of health breastfeeding infants and advised that bacteria for treating infants with diarrhea. Anri Boulardii French microbiologist discovered and isolated Saccharomyces boulardii that was used in South-eastern Asia for thousands of years for treating cholera [14]. Lactobacillus rhamnosus GG strain is one of the most investigated bacteria strain. IT was discovered by two scientists Sherwood Gorbach and Bari Goldin in 1983 [15]. Word probiotic comes from a Greek word pro+bios that means "for life" and it is used for the first time in 1953 when Kollath described organic and nonorganic food additives that are necessary for treating malnutrition. In 1965, Lilly and Still well described probiotics as substances that are produced by one microbe in order to stimulate the growth of another microbe contrary to the term antibiotics.

In 2001, World Health Organization (WAO) defined probiotics as live microbes that can have a positive effects on wellbeing if they use in a proper way and quantities.

In 2002, Food and Agriculture Organization and WHO published recommendation for probiotics in food [16]. In 2014, WHO reviewed probiotic definition in terms of needs for evidence base clinical efficacy of certain probiotics strains. Nowadays, worldwide accepted definition of probiotics is: probiotics are live microbes which benefits and positive effects on human health if they use in adequate quantities are proven in control clinical studies [17, 18]. Old concept of sterile "in utero" development has been abandoned. According to recent studies, colonization of fetal gut started in utero predominantly with maternal oral, vaginal, and gut microbiota. Neither placenta neither amniotic fluid is sterile; fetus received its first dose of probiotics with the ingestion of amniotic fluid [19, 20].

The most relevant prenatal factors for the formation of gut microbiota are maternal hygiene, particularly dental, diet, infectious, and antibiotics usage. Perinatal factors are also antibiotics during delivery, gestational age, the way of delivery, and medical staff in delivery room [21]. Post natal factors include: skin to skin contact, breast feeding, pets, baby bathing, as well as other environmental factors. To summarize all those maternal as well as placental factors have a key role in the development of a child gut microbiota. Moreover, the presence of pathogenic bacteria in amniotic fluid can induce a cascade of inflammatory response and prostaglandin synthesis that leads to the uterus contraction and preterm delivery. In utero infection particularly chorioamnionitis presents key risk factors for preterm delivery.

There is a substantial body of evidence supporting transplacental immune regulation during pregnancy. Maternal IgGs loaded with, for example, microbial components from the mother cross the fetal-maternal barrier by an active process from 13 weeks gestation [22], conveying temporary passive immunity [23] and influencing fetal innate immune development [24]. In contrast, cellular components are generally separated by the placenta, with some leakage in both directions without preference toward a specific cell type [25]. This cellular leakage is functionally important, as maternal cells residing in fetal lymph nodes induce fetal regulatory T cells that suppress antimaternal immunity [26]. Transplacental immune regulation may be further mediated by cytokines and hormones [27], through bacterial products such as short-chain fatty acids or lipopolysaccharides (LPS) [28, 29].

Santner-Nanan et al. have demonstrated a strong correlation of peripheral blood Treg cells between the mother and the fetus [30]. In contrast, there was no significant Treg cell correlation between the father and the fetus, implicating that the specific context of pregnancy, that is, the placental environment, rather than haploidentical genetic parental similarity to the fetus, is responsible for this correlation. Maternal infant alignment in Treg cells appeared to be mediated by IL-10, a pleiotropic cytokine with potent immunoregulatory properties [31]. Treg cells are characterized by increased expression of the IL-10 receptor-α (IL-10RA), making them more sensitive to the effects of IL-10. The IL-10 regulates Bcl-2 expression in Treg cells, which could contribute to Treg cell survival in both the mother and the infant [32].

In the context of alignment between maternal and infant Treg, the evidence that has been studied suggesting an association between complicated pregnancy with preeclampsia and an increased risk of asthma, as well as allergic offspring sensitization [32]. A potential antecedent common to both mother and child is the mother's microbiome and its metabolic products, including short-chain fatty acids (SCFA).

Maternal IgG may play a key role in mediating the association between the maternal microbiome and fetal immune development. Of the five immunoglobulin classes, maternal IgG is the only antibody that significantly crosses the human placenta [22]. The active transport of IgG occurs via the neonatal Fc receptor (FcRn) within the syncytiotrophoblast (ST) cells at the surface of the chorionic villi of the placenta. Once bound to the FcRn receptor, IgG is packaged in endosomes and protected from degradation until it dissociates into the fetal circulation [33, 34].

This materno-fetal IgG transport is an important mechanism that confers passive humoral immunity to the fetus, so that after birth, the infant is protected against infections while its own immune system develops [22, 28]. Allergen-specific maternal IgG also plays a role in the induction of immune tolerance in infant [35]. Until recently, maternal IgG transfer during gestation had only been linked to fetal humoral immunity, but there is now good evidence that maternal IgG also plays a crucial in fetal innate immune development [24]. 61.1% of bacteria isolated in meconium of preterm infants (younger than 33 gestational weeks) are those that are also isolated from amniotic fluid, the majority of them belong to the three strains: Enterobacteria, Enterococcus, Lactobacillus, Photorhabdus, and Tanarella. Those bacteria are found to have a negative correlation with gestational age which suggests their important role in initiation of preterm delivery [36, 37].

4. Gestational age is a second important factor in the development of infant gut microbiota

Studies have been already proven that certain bacteria in amniotic fluid can provoke preterm labor. Preterm babies in comparison to term babies have more anaerobe bacteria. This fact can be described with several facts: preterm babies are at high risk of postnatal complications such as asphyxia, acute respiratory distress development, neonatal sepsis, necrotic enterocolitis, etc. In terms of that they are prescribed more often both oxygen and antibiotics treatment that are together increase hospitalization days particularly in NICU – Neonatal Intensive Care Unit. Only three bacteria strains are found in preterm babies at 10 days of life: Enterobacteria (*E. coli* and *Klebsiella*), Enterococcus faecalis and *Staphylococcus aureus*, and haemolyticus. On the other side, colonization with bifidobacteria in preterm infants is postponed [38]. The way of delivery is the third factor for gut microbiota development. A great number of data suggested that cesarean section alongside with the intrapartal antibiotics usage is independent risk factors for gut disbiosis. During vaginal delivery, an infant become colonize with maternal vaginial bacteria. Grounlad and authors showed that even 6 months after delivery gut of infants born on caesarian section contain less bacteria of Bacteroides fragilis strains. Finland study has proven more bacteria of Clostridium strain in children born on vaginal way in comparison to those born via cesarean section. Lactobacillus, Prevotella, and Sneathia strains are predominant in gut microbiota of children born vaginal way, while on the other side, Staphylococcus, Corynebacterium and Propioni bacterium strains are dominant in another group of children born on caesarian session [39]. Postnatal prevention includes at the first place breast feeding followed with the onetime introduction of solid food and allergens. Breastfed children are proved to have predominantly bifidobacteria strains in their gut microbiota while infants fed with formulas had more bacterioides strains. It is well know that mothers milk contain special ingredients that can have immuno modulation effects on infants immune system. Rutava and authors showed that there is a special interaction between gut microbiota and transforming growth factor beta from human milk that are most potent antiinflammatory factor of a great importance also for maturation of intestinal tract as well as the production of IgA antibodies. According to this hypothesis bacteria from uterus have been actively transported in breast gland and secrete in human milk and in that way transfer immune tolerance to the infants. Moreover, it is proven that if mother use probiotics particularly Lactobacillus strain during breast feeding increase the number of bifidobacteria in gut of breast-fed infants [40].

Intestinal microbiology of early life has been best described in the first thousand days concept (PAI 2014). According to that hypothesis, the first thousand days of early life (230 days prenatal and 2 years postnatal) are crucial for establishing of symbiosis for the whole life. This is one of the most important mechanisms of evolution f as intestinal microbiota is in close relation with etiopathogenesis of allergic, autoimmune disease, and tumors [41].

5. Probiotic in prevention of atopic march

The development of allergic diseases is best described in a concept of atopic march. Allergies start in early infancy with atopic dermatitis, followed by IgE mediated food allergies and asthma development ended up with allergic rhinitis. As we have already mentioned early, intervention is crucial for interrupt atopic march and preventing allergies.

It is very well known for almost 20 years that *Lactobacillus rhamnosus* GG strain 1 × 106 cfu/g given to atopic pregnant women followed with 6 months of postnatal administration to infants can significantly prevent the development of atopic dermatitis at the age of 2 years. Furthermore, protective effects were long lasting for two more years. On the other side, significant increase of atopic dermatitis prevalence has been recorded in the control group in the follow up period [42]. Double blind, randomized, placebo control PandA study investigated the preventive effects of three strains combination Bifidobacterium bifidum W23B (1 × 109 cfg/g), Bifidobacterium lactase W52 (1 × 109 cfu/g) and Lactococcus lactic W58 (1 × 109cfu/l). Administration of this combination to atopic mothers in the last 6 weeks of pregnancy and infants in the first year of life showed preventive effects in the first 3 months of life with the significant changes in intestinal microbiota and decrease in the level of IL-5 production [43]. Those results are in accordance with the results of Zhang meta-analysis who showed that prenatal and postnatal administration of probiotics may reduce the risk of atopic disease in families under risk of allergy and hypersensitivity reaction to food. According to those authors, administration of probiotics to infants born via cesarean section can even benefit more from probiotics [44]. Probiotics are also have positive impact on SCORAD reduction in placebo control study on 27 infants with atopic dermatitis who were breast-fed and received Bifidobacterium lactose Bb-12 1 × 109 cfu/g and Lactobacillus GG 3 × 108 cfu/g in comparison to place group [45]. Majamaa and collaborators showed significant improvement of atopic dermatitis and reduction in fetal concentration of antitripsin-1 and TNF as well as up regulation of Il-10 and down regulation of pro inflammatory cytokines and total IgE antibodies level in infants on hypoallergenic milk formulas who concomitantly received Lactobacillus rhamnosus GG 5 × 108 cfu/g in comparison to placebo group [46]. Pessi's study showed similar Il-10 level improvement in children allergic to cow milk proteins who received Lactobacillus rhamnosus GG 2 × 1010 cfu/g pro doses [47]. Those results are controversial in terms of asthma and wheezing prevention. Two meta-analysis of Elazab and coauthors and Azad and coauthors have failed to prove positive effects of probiotics administration in pregnancy and postnatal on the asthma and wheezing development. Recent meta-analysis of randomized control study of Wei and coauthors did not find enough results to support recommendation of probiotics for asthma prevention in infants [48]. In Filipovic and coauthors study, it is found that *Lactobacillus rhamnosus* GG (LGG) formulation with Zn and vitamin D3 supplementation during the postnatal period (in infancy and early childhood) reduce the severity of atopic dermatitis. Type of delivery, type of feeding breast-feeding versus adapted milk formulas were not found to be statistically associated with risk of atopic dermatitis [49]. According to European Academy for Allergy and Clinical Immunology, there is no official recommendation for probiotic treatment in patients with food allergy [50]. Overall probiotics are proven to have positive effects in primary prevention of allergies even prenatal. According to the results from several studies probiotics have both local and systemic effects. They act locally on the intestinal tract via promoting immune tolerance. Systemically, they act antiinflammatory reducing Th17 response and stimulating TLR and Th1 immune response [51, 52].

6. Conclusion

According to the epidemiological data, allergic diseases have been increasing in the last decades, despite a great variety of effective treatment available. Standard pharmacological treatment of allergies is only symptomatic without the capability to change the natural course of allergic disease. Immunotherapy is the only treatment with the immunomodulatory effects. The second option is probiotics that are not only capable to prevent atopic march but also to prevent the development of allergic disease prenatal. Despite a great number of placebo control randomized studies and meta-analysis, we are still looking for the best probiotic and adequate dose for each level of intervention: prenatal, early postnatal as well as for different manifestation of allergic diseases (atopic dermatitis, food allergies, asthma, and allergic rhinitis).

Author details

Ivana Filipovic[1*], Milan Lackovic[1,2], Slađana Mihajlovic[1,2], Đorđe Filipović[3], Tamara Bakic[4] and Zorica Zivkovic[5,6]

1 Hospital of Gynecology and Obstretics, MC Dr Dragiša Mišović, Belgrade, Serbia

2 School of Medicine, University of Belgrade, Serbia

3 Special Hospital for Cerebrovascular Diseases "Saint Sava", Serbia

4 Faculty of Pharmacy, University of Belgrade, Belgrade, Serbia

5 Children's Hospital for Lung Diseases and Tbc, MC Dr Dragiša Mišović, Belgrade, Serbia

6 Faculty of Pharmacy Novi Sad, Business Academy, Novi Sad, Serbia

*Address all correspondence to: drivanica@yahoo.com

References

[1] Matricardi PM. 99th Dahlem conference on infection, inflammation and chronic inflammatory disorders: Controversial aspects of the 'hygiene hypothesis'. Clinical and Experimental Immunology. 2010;**160**(1):98-105

[2] Prescott S, Allen KJ. Food allergy: Riding the second wave of the allergy epidemic. Pediatric Allergy and Immunology. 2011;**22**(2):155-160. DOI: 10.1111/j.1399-3038.2011.01145.x

[3] Bergmann RL, Bergmann KE, Lau-Schadensdorf S, Luck W, Dannemann A, Bauer CP, et al. Atopic diseases in infancy. The German multicenter atopy study (MAS-90). Pediatric Allergy and Immunology. 1994;**5**:19-25

[4] Holguin F. The atopic march: IgE is not the only road. The Lancet Respiratory Medicine. 2014;**2**:88-90

[5] Gough H, Grabenhenrich L, Reich A, et al. Allergic multimorbidity of asthma, rhinitis and eczema over 20 years in the German birth cohort MAS. Pediatric Allergy and Immunology. 2015;**26**:431-437

[6] Grabenhenrich LB, Gough H, Reich A, Eckers N, Zepp F, Nitsche O, et al. Early-lifedeterminants of asthma from birth to age 20 years: A German birth cohort study. The Journal of Allergy and Clinical Immunology. 2014;**33**:979-988

[7] Caminati M, Duric-Filipovic I, Arasi S, Peroni DG, Zivkovic Z, Senna G. Respiratory allergies in childhood: Recent advances and future challenges. Pediatric Allergy and Immunology. December 2015;**26**(8): 702-710. DOI: 10.1111/pai.12509

[8] Hayward AR. The human fetus and newborn: Development of the immune response. Birth Defects Original Article Series. 1983;**19**(3):289-294

[9] Halken S. Prevention of allergic disease in childhood: Clinical and epidemiological aspects of primary and secondary allergy prevention. Pediatric Allergy and Immunology. 2004;**15**(Suppl 16):9-32

[10] Illi S, Weber J, Zutavern A, et al. Perinatal influences on the development of asthma and atopy in childhood. Annals of Allergy, Asthma & Immunology. February 2014;**112**(2):132-139

[11] Herbst T, Sichelstiel A, Schär C, Yadava K, Bürki K, Cahenzli J, et al. Dysregulation of allergic airway inflammation in the absence of microbial colonization. American Journal of Respiratory and Critical Care Medicine. 2011;**184**(2):198-205

[12] von Mutius E, Vercelli D. Farm living: Effects on childhood asthma and allergy. Nature Reviews. Immunology. 2010;**10**(12):861-868

[13] Ege MJ, Mayer M, Normand AC, Genuneit J, Cookson WO, Braun-Fahrländer C, et al. Exposure to environmental microorganisms and childhood asthma. The New England Journal of Medicine. 2011

[14] Schrezenmeir J, de Vrese M. Probiotics, prebiotics, and synbiotics--approaching a definition. The American Journal of Clinical Nutrition. 2001;**73** (2 Suppl):361S-364S. DOI: 10.1093/ajcn/73.2.361s

[15] Conway PL, Gorbach SL, Goldin BR. Survival of lactic acid bacteria in the human stomach and adhesion to intestinal cells. Journal of Dairy Science. 1987;**70**(1):1-12

[16] Živković Z, Filipović I, Filipović Đ. Probiotics for acute gastroenteritis – pediatrician's thinking and decision. Preventive Pediatric. 2020;**6**(1-2):9-11

[17] Guidelines for the Evaluation of Probiotics in Food. Available from: www.who.int/foodsafty/fs_managment/en/probiotic_guidelines.pdf [Accessed: April 2020]

[18] Hill C, Guarner F, Reid G, Gibson GR, Merenstein DJ, Pot B, et al. Expert consensus document. The international scientific Association for Probiotics and Prebiotics consensus statement on the scope and appropriate use of the term probiotic. Nature Reviews. Gastroenterology & Hepatology. 2014;**11**(8):506-514. DOI: 10.1038/nrgastro.2014.66

[19] Perez-Muñoz ME, Arrieta MC, Ramer-Tait AE, Walter J. A critical assessment of the "sterile womb" and "in utero colonization" hypotheses: Implications for research on the pioneer infant microbiome. Microbiome. 2017;**5**(1):48. DOI: 10.1186/s40168-017-0268-4

[20] Aagaard K, Ma J, Antony KM, Ganu R, Petrosino J, Versalovic J. The placenta harbors a unique microbiome. Science Translational Medicine. 2014;**6**(237):237-265. DOI: 10.1126/scitranslmed.3008599

[21] Teshome A, Yitayeh A. Relationship between periodontal disease and preterm low birth weight: Systematic review. The Pan African Medical Journal. 2016;**24**:215

[22] Palmeira P, Quinello C, Silveira-Lessa AL, et al. IgG placental transfer in healthy and pathological pregnancies. Clinical & Developmental Immunology. Hindawi Publishing Corporation Clinical and Developmental Immunology. Vol. 2012. 2012. Article ID 98564. p. 13. DOI: 10.1155/2012/985646

[23] Firan M, Bawdon R, Radu C, et al. The MHC class I-related receptor, FcRn, plays an essential role in the maternofetal transfer of gamma-globulin in humans. International Immunology. 2001;**13**:993-1002

[24] Gomez de Agüero M, Ganal-Vonarburg SC, Fuhrer T, et al. The maternal microbiota drives early postnatal innate immune development. Science. 2016;**351**:1296-1302

[25] Loubière LS, Lambert NC, Flinn LJ, et al. Maternal microchimerism in healthy adults in lymphocytes, monocyte/macrophages and NK cells. Laboratory Investigation. 2006;**86**:1185-1192

[26] Mold JE, Michaëlsson J, Burt TD, et al. Maternal alloantigens promote the development of tolerogenic fetal regulatory T cells in utero. Science. 2008;**322**:1562-1565

[27] Lacković M, Mihajlović S, Bakić T, Marina L, Stefan Šojat A, Ilić M, et al. Imunski sistem u trudnoći. Preventive Pediatric. 2020;**6**(1-2):37-40

[28] Thorburn AN, McKenzie CI, Shen S, et al. Evidence that asthma is a developmental origin disease influenced by maternal diet and bacterial metabolites. Nature Communications. 2015;**6**:7320

[29] Voltolini C, Battersby S, Etherington SL, et al. A novel antiinflammatory role for the short-chain fatty acids in human labor. Endocrinology. 2012;**153**:395-403

[30] Conrad ML, Ferstl R, Teich R, et al. Maternal TLR signaling is required for prenatal asthma protection by the nonpathogenic microbe Acinetobacter lwoffii F78. The Journal of Experimental Medicine. 2009;**206**:2869-2877

[31] Santner-Nanan B, Straubinger K, Hsu P, et al. Fetal-maternal alignment of regulatory T cells correlates with IL-10 and Bcl-2 upregulation in pregnancy. Journal of Immunology. 2013;**191**:145-153

[32] Mosser DM, Zhang X. Interleukin-10: New perspectives on an

old cytokine. Immunological Reviews. 2008;**226**:205-218

[33] Kumpel BM, Manoussaka MS. Placental immunology and maternal alloimmune responses. Vox Sanguinis. 2012;**102**:2-12

[34] Schneider H, Miller RK. Receptor-mediated uptake and transport of macromolecules in the human placenta. The International Journal of Developmental Biology. 2010;**54**:367-375

[35] Shreiner A, Huffnagle GB, Noverr MC. The "microflora hypothesis" of allergic disease. Advances in Experimental Medicine and Biology. 2008;**635**:113-134

[36] Ardissone AN, de la Cruz DM, Davis-Richardson AG, et al. Meconium microbiome analysis identifies bacteria correlated with premature birth. PLoS One. 2014;**9**(3):e90784

[37] Magne F, Suau A, Pochart P, Desleux JF. Fecal microbial community in preterm infants. Journal of Pediatric Gastroenterology and Nutrition. 2005;**41**:386-392

[38] Arboleya S, Sánchez B, Solís G, et al. Impact of prematurity and perinatal antibiotics on the developing intestinal microbiota: A functional inference study. International Journal of Molecular Sciences. 2016;**17**(5):649

[39] Grönlund MM, Lehtonen OP, Eerola E, Kero P. Fecal microflora in healthy infants born by different methods of delivery: Permanent changes in intestinal flora after cesarean delivery. Journal of Pediatric Gastroenterology and Nutrition. 1999;**28**(1):19-25

[40] Rautava S, Luoto R, Salminen S, Isolauri E. Microbial contact during pregnancy, intestinal colonization and human disease. Nature Reviews. Gastroenterology & Hepatology. 2012;**9**(10):565-576

[41] Wopereis H, Oozeer R, Knipping K, Belzer C, Knol J. The first thousand days - intestinal microbiology of early life: Establishing a symbiosis. Pediatric Allergy and Immunology. 2014;**25**(5):428-438. DOI: 10.1111/pai.12232

[42] Kalliomaki M, Salminen S, Arvilommi H, Pentti K, Pertti K, Isolauri E. Probiotics in primary prevention of atopic disease: A randomised placebo- controlled trial. Lancet. 2001;**357**:1076-1079

[43] Niers L, Martín R, Rijkers G, Sengers F, Timmerman H, van Uden N, et al. The effects of selected probiotic strains on the development of eczema (the PandA study). Allergy. 2009;**64**(9):1349-1358

[44] Zhang G-Q, Hu H-J, Liu C-Y, Zhang Q, Shakya S, Le Z-Y. Probiotics for prevention of atopy and food hypersensitivity in early childhood. Medicine. 2016;**95**(8):e2562

[45] Isolauri E, Arvola T, Sutas Y, Moilanen E, Salminen S. Probiotics in the management of atopic eczema. Clinical and Experimental Allergy. 2000;**30**:1604-1610

[46] Majamaa H, Isolauri E. Probiotics: A novel approach in the management of food allergy. The Journal of Allergy and Clinical Immunology. 1997;**99**:179-185

[47] Pessi T, Sutas Y, Hurme M, Isolauri E. Interleu-kin-10 generation in atopic children following oral Lactobacillus rhamnosus GG. Clinical and Experimental Allergy. 2000;**30**:1804-1808

[48] Azad MB, Coney JG, Kozyrskyj AL, Field CJ, Ramsey CD, Backer AB, et al. Probiotic supplementation during

pregnancy or infancy for the prevention of asthma and wheeze: Systematic review and meta-analysis. BMJ. 2013;**347**:f6471

[49] Filipovic I, Ostojic O, Vekovic V, Lackovic M, Zivkovic Z. Combination of Lactobacillus Rhamnosus LGG, vitamin D3 and Zn in preventing atopic dermatitis in infancy. American Journal of Pediatrics. 2020;**6**(3):280-284. DOI: 10.11648/j.ajp.20200603.26

[50] Muraro A, Halken S, Arshad SH, Beyer K, Dubois AE, Du Toit G, et al. EAACI food allergy and anaphylaxis guidelines. Primary prevention of food allergy. Allergy. 2014;**69**(5):590-601

[51] Ozdemir O. Various effects of different probiotic strains in allergic disorders: An update from laboratory and clinical data. Clinical and Experimental Immunology. 2010;**160**(3):295-304

[52] Özdemir Ö. Any benefits of probiotics in allergic disorders? Allergy and Asthma Proceedings. 2009;**31**:103-111

Chapter 8

Biologicals in Atopic Dermatitis

Suvarna Samudrala

Abstract

Atopic dermatitis (AD) is a debilitating condition, and its management in both children and adults can be challenging for clinicians and patients alike. The current treatment options approved by the Food and Drug Administration (FDA) have variable efficacies, and long-term adverse effects, which further complicate the plan of management. There has been considerable progress towards the use of targeted medicines like biologicals and small molecular agents for atopic dermatitis. Various molecules targeting the TH2 pathway, JAK/STAT pathway, cAMP, IL-22, Il-12/IL-23 and IgE, have been developed, and are being studied extensively in both adults and pediatric patients of atopic dermatitis. Currently, only Dupilumab is approved by the FDA for the treatment of moderate to severe refractory atopic dermatitis. The other biological agents are currently in phase 2 or phase 3 trials. There is a paucity of multicentric, large-scale studies on the above drugs, along with a lack of comparative studies with the existing modalities of treatment. Therefore, more studies with a larger sample size and longer follow up periods are needed to determine their efficacy and long-term safety profiles. Overall, these agents are likely to be a part of the therapeutic armamentarium for atopic dermatitis in the near future.

Keywords: atopic dermatitis, biologicals, Dupilumab, Th2 pathway, JAK/STAT pathway

1. Introduction

Atopic dermatitis (AD) is a debilitating condition, and its management in both children and adults can be challenging for clinicians and patients alike. About 20% of patients with AD manifest with moderate to severe forms of the disease, which are refractory to conventional treatment. The current treatment options approved by the Food and Drug Administration (FDA) have variable efficacies, and long-term adverse effects, which further complicate the plan of management [1].

There has been considerable progress towards the use of targeted medicines like biologicals and small molecular agents to block specific cytokines, their receptors, or transcription factors. The indications for these agents are also rapidly expanding, from adults to the pediatric population. Their formulations range from injections to oral tablets, and topical creams and ointments [2].

Advances in understanding the various immunopathological changes occurring in atopic dermatitis have allowed the identification of various therapeutic molecular targets and synthesis of various biological agents [1].

IntechOpen

2. Classification of biological agents (based on their mechanism of action)

1. IgE directed therapy-Omalizumab

2. Th2 inhibitors:

   - Anti IL-4-Dupilumab

   - Anti IL-4/IL-13 agents-Lebrikizumab, Tralokinumab

   - IL-31 directed therapy-Nemolizumab

3. Anti IL-12/23 agents-Ustekinumab

4. IL-22 blockade-Fezakinumab

5. Thymic stromal lymphopoietin directed therapy-Tezepelumab

6. JAK inhibitors-Tofacitinib, Abrocitinib, Delgocitinib, Upadacitinib, Ruxolitinib, Baricitinib

7. Miscellaneous agents

2.1 IgE directed therapy-Omalizumab

Omalizumab is a recombinant humanized monoclonal IgG1 antibody, which has been approved by the FDA for the treatment of moderate to severe persistent asthma and chronic spontaneous urticaria. It has also been shown to be beneficial in chronic inducible urticaria, allergic rhinitis, eosinophilic esophagitis, food allergy, anaphylaxis, as premedication in allergen specific immunotherapy, Churg-Strauss disease, eosinophilic otitis media, allergic bronchopulmonary aspergillosis, chronic rhinosinusitis, bullous pemphigoid, contact dermatitis and atopic dermatitis [1].

Mechanism of action

It is composed of 5% murine and 95% human sequence. Omalizumab combines with the free, soluble IgE, blocking its binding to its receptors, and subsequently preventing allergen-induced mediator release.

It dramatically reduces the serum levels of free IgE (by 99% in the first two hours after administration), which then downregulates the expression of IgE high-affinity receptors on immune cells. It also decreases the expression of several cytokines (such as IL-5, 8, 13) and inhibits the recruitment of immune cells (T-cells, eosinophils, and macrophages) to the affected sites. Therefore, it inhibits both the immediate and the late inflammatory phases. It is also involved in apoptosis of mast cells and eosinophils.

Omalizumab in AD

Anti-IgE therapy in AD has shown conflicting results. Although most data from small randomized trials, case series and case reports documented clinical benefit and resolution of eczema, a small number of studies showed no improvement of disease with Omalizumab. Filaggrin mutations and raised serum IgE levels were associated with a poorer response to Omalizumab [3]. All of the studies noted the safety profile in both adult and pediatric population treated with Omalizumab. However, the variable response to treatment and lack of standardized dosing protocols remain major drawbacks. Another notable conclusion of placebo-controlled studies showed no significant improvement with Omalizumab compared to the control groups [1].

2.2 TH2 inhibitors

2.2.1 Anti IL-4 (Dupilumab)

Dupilumab was approved by the FDA in 2017 for the treatment of adults with moderate to severe refractory atopic dermatitis [1]. It was further approved in 2020 for children aged 6 to 11 years with moderate-to-severe atopic dermatitis [4]. Currently, it is the only biological approved for the treatment of AD.

Dose—It is available as prefilled syringes containing 300 mg Or 200 mg of the drug

- Adults and children (6–11 years weighing >60 kgs): Loading dose of 600 mg subcutaneously followed by 300 mg every 2 weeks

- Pediatric patients (weight > 30-<60 kgs)-400 mg s/c loading dose followed by 200 mg every 2 weeks

- Pediatric patients (weight > 15-<30 kgs)-Loading dose of 600 mg subcutaneously followed by 300 mg every 4 weeks

Mechanism of action

Both IL-4 and IL-13 are key drivers of the Th2-mediated allergic inflammation. They synergistically act via a common receptor, IL-4Rα, to activate the signaling proteins [signal transducer and activator of transcription 6 (STAT6) and Janus kinase-1 (JAK1)]. IL-4 induces the immunoglobulin isotype class switch to IgE, promotes the Th2 phenotype, prevents T-cell apoptosis, renders the T-cells refractory to corticosteroids, and induces the expression of VCAM-1 on endothelial cells, subsequently promoting the recruitment of T-cells, eosinophils, basophils and monocytes. Gene polymorphisms in IL-4, IL – 13 and IL-4Rα have been associated with AD in certain populations.[1] In the presence of IL-4 and IL-13, keratinocytes exhibit significantly less FLG gene expression, leading to epidermal barrier dysfunction. Dupilumab is a fully humanized monoclonal antibody against interleukin-4 (IL-4) receptor-α (IL-4Rα) [5].

Dupilumab in AD

Dupilumab has been a major addition to the therapeutic armamentarium of moderate to severe refractory AD.

Administration of dupilumab leads to the following molecular changes:

1. downregulation of markers of epidermal proliferation

2. downregulation of inflammatory mediators

3. upregulation of structural proteins

4. upregulation of lipid metabolism proteins

5. upregulation of epidermal barrier proteins resulting in normalization of skin.

6. Reduction in genes activating T cells

7. reduction in serum levels of CCL17 (or thymus and activation-regulated chemokine), a key regulator of Th2-mediated immunity and a specific biomarker of AD disease activity [6].

Mono-therapy or combined therapy with Dupilumab has shown to be beneficial in the effective control of disease, improvement in skin lesions, significant reduction in pruritus and an improved quality of life of affected patients. Studies have shown that the transcriptome of skin lesions of AD resembled that of the non-lesional skin after only 4 weeks of treatment with Dupilumab. Many clinical trials investigating the efficacy and safety of Dupilumab in AD have shown a rapid and marked improvement of disease activity, and a safe profile of administration [1].

A phase 3 trial [7] conducted in 251 adolescents showed statistically significant improvement in the signs, symptoms, and quality of life after 16 weeks of Dupilumab injection, with the 2-weekly regimen showing a better response.

In pediatric patients, a multi-centre review [8] done on 111 children showed ≥2 point improvement in the Investigator Global Assessment (IGA) score in 64.3% patients after 9 weeks.

The mean dosage used in children was 8.7 mg/kg loading dose followed by 5.1 mg/kg maintenance dose every other week.

Adverse effects reported include worsening of alcohol flushing; new regional dermatitis in face, conjunctivitis and eosinophilia have been reported with Dupilumab [9, 10].

2.2.2 Anti Il-4/Il-13 agents: Lebrikizumab and Tralokinumab

IL-13 is overexpressed in the skin lesions of AD patients and appears to negatively regulate the expression of genes encoding crucial structural proteins (such as loricrin, involucrin), leading to be the impairment of the epidermal barrier. Lebrikizumab and Tralokinumab selectively target IL-13 and prevent the formation of the IL-13Rα1/IL-4Rα heterodimer receptor signaling complex [11]. Significant clinical improvement has been seen in moderate to severe AD in a small number of Phase 2 studies, with a good safety profile. However, concomitant topical corticosteroid therapy in enrolled patients limits data regarding their efficacy. Therefore, further studies are needed to confirm their beneficial effects in AD [1]. It is currently in Phase 3 trials. It is given subcutaneously every 4 weeks, but its effective dose is yet to be determined [12].

2.2.3 IL-31 directed therapy: Nemolizumab

It is a humanized monoclonal antibody against IL-31 receptor A. IL-31 is expressed predominantly by Th2 lymphocytes, functions to target keratinocytes, epithelial cells, eosinophils, basophils and monocytes. It is overexpressed in AD skin lesions [13]. A phase 3 randomized, double blind, placebo-controlled clinical trial [14] noted a significant clinical improvement profile in adult patients with refractory moderate to severe AD, as compared to the placebo group. However, the duration of the study was only for 16 weeks. Further studies are needed to confirm long-term efficacy and safety profile. The maximum efficacy has been seen with 60 mg subcutaneous injections given every 4 weeks.

2.3 Anti IL-12/IL-23 agent: Ustekinumab

Ustekinumab is a human immunoglobulin G1κ monoclonal antibody against the common p40-subunit shared by IL-12 and – 23. IL-23 is responsible for Th17 cell development, and is associated with tissue damage in several inflammatory conditions. IL-23 levels positively correlates with the severity of atopic dermatitis among children. Results regarding the utility of Ustekinumab in the treatment of AD brought inconclusive results. While several case reports have suggested the efficacy of Ustekinumab in severe AD, some others show a moderate effect or a lack of it. This may be due to the multifactorial aetiopathology of the disease. Recently, Noda et al. [1] showed a predominant Th17 immune pattern in Asian AD patients. Such data is valuable for identifying individuals who are most likely to benefit from therapy. Further studies are needed to determine its efficacy and safety and the treatment of AD.

2.4 IL-22 blocker: Fezakinumab

IL-22 promotes epidermal hyperplasia and skin barrier dysfunction in AD. Fezankinumab is an anti IL-22 antibody. Phase 2 placebo-controlled studies have shown progressive and sustained clinical improvement of moderate-to-severe AD after 12 weeks of treatment. It is given intravenously with a loading dose of 600 mg followed by 300 mg every 2 weeks [1, 15].

2.5 Thymic stromal lymphopoietin directed therapy

TSLP is a pivotal pro-inflammatory cytokine in both acute and chronic skin lesions of AD. Tezepelumab is a human monoclonal antibody that prevents the interaction of thymic stromal lymphopoietin (TSLP) with its receptor [1]. Phase 2a trials [16] using 280 mg subcutaneous injections every 2 weeks showed an insignificant improvement in the EASI and SCORAD values after 12 weeks of treatment. Therefore, it is unlikely to be a major treatment option in the near future.

2.6 JAK inhibitors

Targeting of the Janus kinase (JAK) and spleen tyrosine kinase (SYK) pathways attenuates signaling via multiple immune pathways (Th1, Th2, Th17 and Th22) and enhances keratinocyte differentiation [17]. Although these drugs have emerged as promising treatment options for AD, their long-term safety profiles are yet to be determined [4].

Tofacitinib shows specificity for JAK3, baricitinib mainly inhibits JAK1 and JAK2, upadacitinib, ruxolitinib and abrocitinib are selective for JAK1. Delgocitinib inhibits JAK1, JAK2 and JAK3. At present, baricitinib and upadacitinib are also at the final stages of clinical development for atopic dermatitis [18].

2.6.1 Tofacitinib

The first JAK inhibitor to be studied in humans, has been developed in both topical and oral formulations, although only oral tofacitinib is commercially available [4]. A single phase 2a randomized, double-blind, vehicle-controlled study on 69 adults with mild-to-moderate AD showed significant improvement(−81.7% vs. −29.9%) in the EASI score after 4 weeks of applying 2% tofacitinb ointment [19, 20].

2.6.2 Delgocitinib

0.025% and 0.5% ointment has shown encouraging results in recent Phase 3 [21] studies in adult patients, and Phase 2a studies [22] in pediatric patients with moderate to severe AD up to 4 weeks and 28 weeks respectively, with no serious side effects

2.6.3 Oral Abrocitinib

Oral Abrocitinib was evaluated in a phase 3 double-blind placebo-controlled trial, [23] and was effective and well tolerated in adolescents and adults with moderate-to-severe atopic dermatitis. In this trial, 387 patients (aged ≥12 years; 43% women) with moderate-to-severe atopic dermatitis (60% with moderate disease; 40% with severe disease) were randomly assigned (2:2:1) to receive oral abrocitinib 100 mg, 200 mg, or placebo once a day. At week 12, 37 (24%) of 156 patients in the abrocitinib 100 mg group and 67 (44%) of 154 patients in the abrocitinib 200 mg group had achieved an Investigator Global Assessment response of clear or almost clear (score 0–1) compared with six (8%) of 77 patients in the placebo group, and 62 (40%) of 156 patients in the abrocitinib 100 mg group and 96 (62%) of 154 patients in the abrocitinib 200 mg group achieved a 75% improvement or more in Eczema Area and Severity Index (EASI) score from baseline, compared with nine (12%) of 77 patients in the placebo group. This seems to be a promising future option for AD.

2.6.4 Baricitinib

Phase 2 RCT [24] in 124 adults with 2 mg and 4 mg qd dose of Baricitinib showed significant reduction in pruritus and inflammation after 16 weeks. The common adverse effects noted were headache, increased creatine phosphokinase levels and nasopharyngitis.

2.6.5 Ruxolitinib

Phase 2 RCT was conducted in 252 adults with AD, to study the efficacy of 0.15% cream qd, 0.5% RUX cream qd, 1.5% RUX cream qd and 1.5% RUX cream bid. The study showed significant symptomatic improvement after 4 weeks of application, which was sustained for 12 weeks, with good tolerability and no major adverse effects [19, 25].

2.7 Miscellaneous

Studies with the following drugs have either failed to demonstrate a significant improvement or are currently under phase 2 trials:

- Mepolizumab-a humanized monoclonal anti-IL-5 antibody
- Rituximab - a chimeric monoclonal antibody against CD20
- Tumor necrosis-α factor/receptor (TNF-α) inhibitors such as Infliximab, Etanercept, and Adalimumab.
- High-dose intravenous immunoglobulins (IVIGs)
- Anti IL-17: Secukinumab

- Anti IL-6: Tocilizumab
- Recombinant human interferon-γ (rhIFN-γ)
- Natural AhR (therapeutic aryl hydrocarbon receptor) modulating agent: Tapinarof
- T-cell modulating agents (Efalizumab and Alefacept) [1]
- Anti IL-1α-Bermekimab [26].

3. Conclusion

Biologicals offer exciting prospects in the future management strategies for atopic dermatitis. However, the paucity of multicentric, large-scale, randomized trials, a high cost of treatment, along with a lack of comparative studies with the existing modalities of treatment are the major obstacles to their large scale use in clinical practice. Therefore, more studies with a larger sample size and longer follow up periods are needed to determine their efficacy and long-term safety profiles. Although Dupilumab is currently the only biological drug approved by the FDA for atopic dermatitis, other biologicals have also shown promising results and are expected to be a major part of the therapeutic armamentarium for atopic dermatitis in the near future.

Author details

Suvarna Samudrala
Lady Hardinge Medical College, New Delhi, India

*Address all correspondence to: chuvvi89@gmail.com

References

[1] Deleanu D, Nedelea I. Biological therapies for atopic dermatitis: An update (review). Experimental and Therapeutic Medicine. 2019;**17**:1061-1067

[2] Ahn K, Kim BE, Kim J, Leung DY. Recent advances in atopic dermatitis. Current Opinion in Immunology. 2020;**66**:14-21

[3] Del Rosso JQ. More from the pipeline of clinical research on SELECTED SYSTEMIC THERAPIES FOR ATOPIC DERMATITIS. The Journal of Clinical and Aesthetic Dermatology. 2019;**12**(5):49-53

[4] Barrett, J. FDA Approves Dupilumab for Atopic Dermatitis in Children. Retrieved May 26, 2020, from https://www.drugtopics.com/autoimmune-diseases/fda-approves-dupilumab-atopic-dermatitis-children.

[5] Gooderham MJ, Hong HC, Eshtiaghi P, Papp KA. Dupilumab: A review of its use in the treatment of atopic dermatitis. Journal of the American Academy of Dermatology. 2018;**78**:S28-S36

[6] Wu J, Guttman-Yassky E. Efficacy of biologics in atopic dermatitis. **Expert Opinion on Biological Therapy**. 2020;**20**:525-538

[7] Simpson EL, Paller AS, Siegfried EC, Boguniewicz M, Sher L, Gooderham MJ, et al. Efficacy and safety of Dupilumab in adolescents with uncontrolled moderate to severe atopic dermatitis: A phase 3 randomized clinical trial. JAMA Dermatology. 2020;**156**(1):44-56

[8] Igelman S, Kurta AO, Sheikh U, McWilliams A, Armbrecht E, Jackson Cullison SR, et al. Off-label use of dupilumab for pediatric patients with atopic dermatitis: A multicenter retrospective review. Journal of the American Academy of Dermatology. 2020;**82**:407-411

[9] Giavina-Bianchi M, Rizzo LV, Giavina-Bianchi P. Severe atopic dermatitis: Dupilumab is not just safer. but more efficient. Allergol Immunopathol (Madr). 2020;**1118**. Available from. DOI: https://doi.org/10.1016/j.aller.2019.12.005

[10] Faiz S, Giovanelli J, Podevin C, Jachiet M, Bouaziz JD, Reguiai Z, et al. Effectiveness and safety of dupilumab for the treatment of atopic dermatitis in a real-life French multicenter adult cohort. Journal of the American Academy of Dermatology. 2019;**81**:143-151

[11] Guttman-Yassky E, Blauvelt A, Eichenfield LF, et al. Efficacy and safety of Lebrikizumab, a high-affinity interleukin 13 inhibitor, in adults with moderate to severe atopic dermatitis: A phase 2b randomized clinical trial. JAMA Dermatology. 2020;**156**(4):411-420

[12] Wollenberg A, Howell MD, Guttman-Yassky E, Silverberg JI, Kell C, Ranade K, et al. Treatment of atopic dermatitis with tralokinumab, an anti–IL-13 mAb. The Journal of Allergy and Clinical Immunology. 2019;**143**:135-141

[13] Silverberg JI, Pinter A, Pulka G, Poulin Y, Bouaziz JD, Reguiai Z, et al. Phase 2B randomized study of nemolizumab in adults with moderate-to-severe atopic dermatitis and severe pruritus. The Journal of Allergy and Clinical Immunology. 2020;**145**:173-182

[14] Kabashima K, Matsumura T, Komazaki H, Kawashima M. Trial of Nemolizumab and topical agents for atopic dermatitis with pruritus. The New England Journal of Medicine. 2020;**383**:141-150

[15] Guttman-Yassky E, Brunner PM, Neumann AU, Traidl-Hoffmann C, Krueger JG, Lebwohl MG. Efficacy and safety of Fezakinumab (an IL-22 monoclonal antibody) in adults with moderate-to-severe atopic dermatitis inadequately controlled by conventional treatments: A randomized, double-blind. phase 2a trial. 2018;**78**:872-881

[16] Simpson EL, Parnes JR, She D, Crouch S, Rees W, Mo M, et al. Tezepelumab, an anti-thymic stromal lymphopoietin monoclonal antibody, in the treatment of moderate to severe atopic dermatitis: A randomized phase 2a clinical trial. Journal of the American Academy of Dermatology. 2019;**80**:1013-1021

[17] He H, Guttman-Yassky EJAK. Inhibitors for atopic dermatitis: An. Update. 2019;**20**:181-192

[18] Weidinger S. Schreiber S. Abrocitinib for atopic dermatitis: a step forward. 2020;**396**:215-217

[19] Del Rosso JQ. An update on the latest developments in nonsteroidal topical therapy for atopic dermatitis. The Journal of Clinical and Aesthetic Dermatology. 2020;**13**(5):44-48

[20] Bissonnette R, Papp KA, Poulin Y, Gooderham M, Raman M, et al. Topical tofacitinib for atopic dermatitis: A phase IIa randomized trial. The British Journal of Dermatology. 2016 Nov;**175**(5):902-911

[21] Nakagawa H, Nemoto O, Igarashi A, Saeki H, Kaino H, Nagata T. Delgocitinib ointment, a topical Janus kinase inhibitor, in adult patients with moderate to severe atopic dermatitis: A phase 3, randomized, double-blind, vehicle-controlled study and an open-label, long-term extension study. Journal of the American Academy of Dermatology. 2020;**82**:823-831

[22] Nakagawa H, Nemoto O, Igarashi A, Saeki H, Oda M, Kabashima K, et al. Phase 2 clinical study of delgocitinib ointment in pediatric patients with atopic dermatitis. The Journal of Allergy and Clinical Immunology. 2019;**144**(6):1575-1583

[23] Simpson EL, Sinclair R, Forman S, Wollenberg A, Achoff R, Cork M, et al. Efficacy and safety of abrocitinib in adults and adolescents with moderate-to-severe atopic dermatitis (JADE MONO-1): A multicentre, double-blind, randomised, placebo-controlled, phase 3 trial. Lancet. 2020;**396**:255-266

[24] Guttman-Yassky E, Silverberg JI, Nemoto O, Forman SB, Wilke A, Prescilla R, et al. Baricitinib in adult patients with moderate-to-severe atopic dermatitis: A phase 2 parallel, double-blinded, randomized placebo-controlled multiple-dose study. Journal of the American Academy of Dermatology. 2019;**80**:913-921

[25] Kim BS, Howell MD, Sun K, Papp K, Nasir A, Kuligowski ME. Treatment of atopic dermatitis with ruxolitinib cream (JAK1/JAK2 inhibitor) or triamcinolone cream. The Journal of Allergy and Clinical Immunology. 2020;**145**:572-582

[26] Wu J, Guttman-Yassky E. Efficacy of biologics in atopic dermatitis. **Expert Opin Biol Ther** 2020. Available from DOI: 10.1080/14712598.2020.1722998.